From Flab to Fab in 8 Weeks

Busy Mom's

GUIDE TO A LEANER BODY AND HEALTHY EATING

by Allison Jackson

Dedicated to Scott,
Connor and Madison

TABLE OF CONTENTS

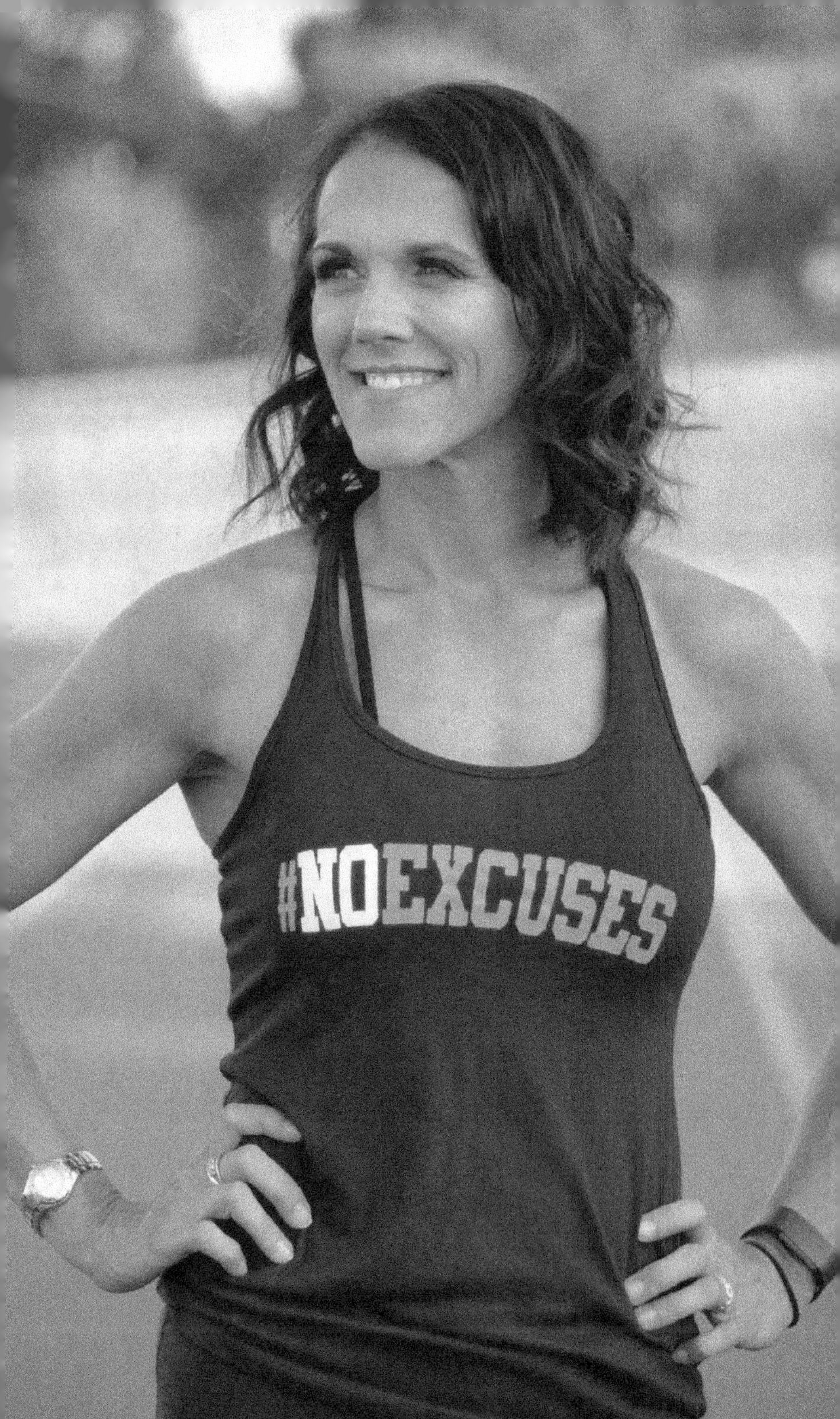
#NOEXCUSES

My Story

Losing weight feels like it's been a lifelong battle for me. I can vividly remember trying my first diet in the 7th grade at around 12 years old. I ate one meal and starved myself the rest of the day. Needless to say, that was neither a healthy nor sustainable diet…and I lasted on that for about a day.

Since that time, I've pretty much tried every diet under the sun: The Zone Diet, The South Beach Diet, Atkins, Weight Watchers. You name it, I've tried it. Each time, I would lose a few pounds and gain double that amount back. I gained the "Freshman 15" in college. I gained 40 pounds with each pregnancy. Somehow, I managed to lose those pounds, but never really felt good in my own skin. I didn't have a body that made me feel good about myself or how I looked. I was self-conscious in a bathing suit. I hated clothes shopping. I wanted to be a different size and a much lower weight, but it felt like I was chasing some magical unicorn. I developed a love-hate (mostly hate) relationship with my scale.

Now mind you, I have been passionate about fitness since I was 13 years old. I took Jazzercise classes with my mom, then taught aerobics in college, which evolved into running 5ks and doing sprint triathlons in my early 20s.

Then, I upped the ante and ran two marathons (Philadelphia and New York City) in my early 30s. After conquering those goals, I finally achieved my bucket-list goal of competing in a figure competition (think bodybuilding meets beauty pageant) at the ripe old age of 38. This led to my love affair with weight training. (I had always enjoyed it, but competing took my lifting program to a whole new level.)

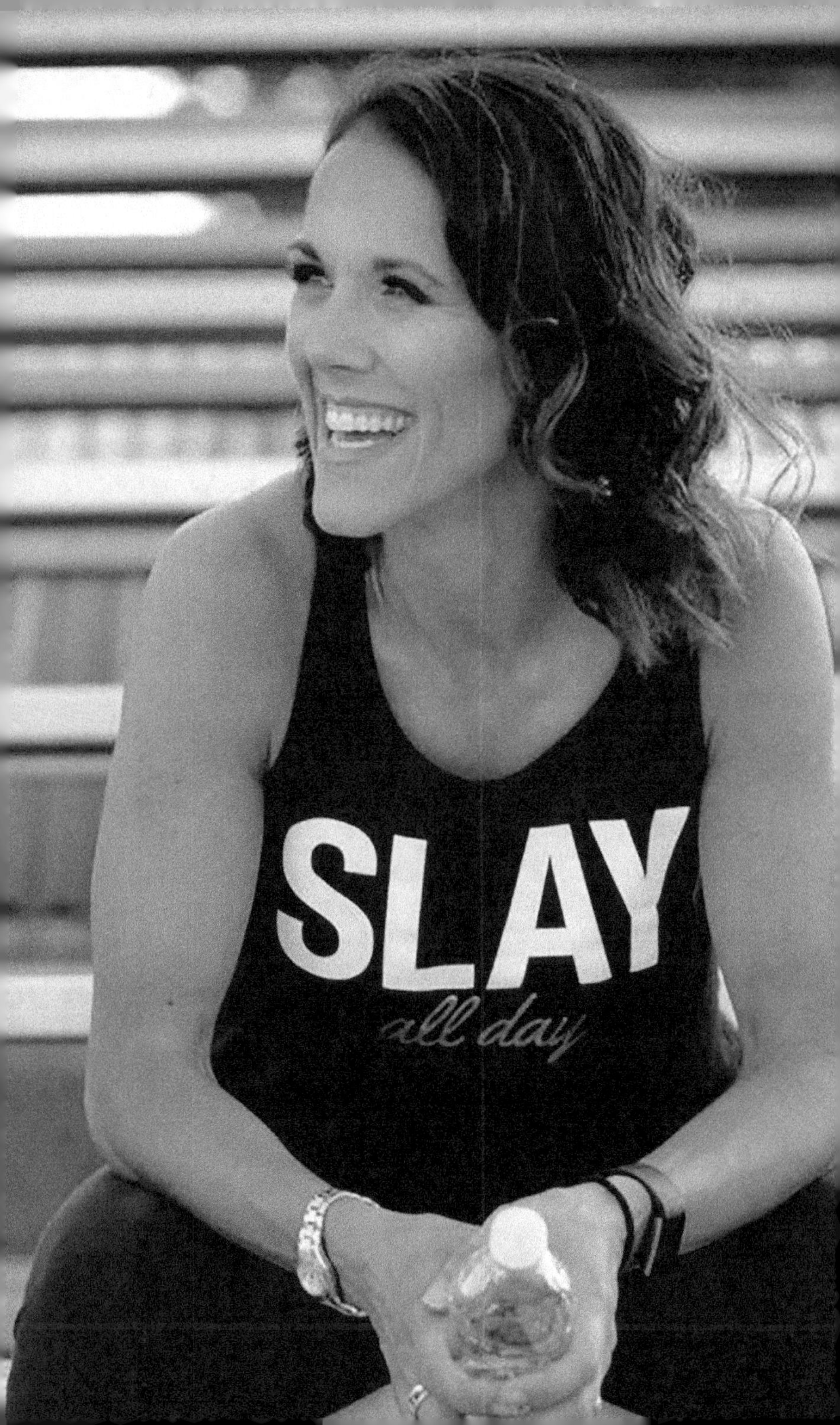

SLAY
all day

As I progressed and performed increasingly better in my competitions, more and more people started to ask me how I was able to drop body fat and hit the stage each year. Year after year, I would drop 15 or more pounds within the course of four to five months. It was done without starvation or crazy foods, but by tracking my macros, eating nutritious food and doing effective workouts. I began coaching others and teaching them what I learned. As my clients started dropping weight, I felt absolutely incredible to be able to help people in this way. Coaching has been such an amazing experience for me that I couldn't wait to help more people! The more people I help, the more it lights me up! My goal is to help as many people as I possibly can, which is one of the many reasons for writing this book.

What you'll find in this book is all of the things I've learned over the course of my competing career, coupled with coaching my clients using my eight-week program. If you follow what I've outlined, you can expect an entire transformation. In addition to losing weight, you will have a newfound confidence. Your clothes will fit better. You'll have more energy. People will begin to tell you that you look like you lost weight. You will sleep better and look forward to being active. The way you approach food will be completely altered and you won't stress out about holidays, traveling, or social gatherings. You will know exactly how to approach each scenario. Are you ready to finally learn how to get your best body once and for all?

Allison Jackson Fitness

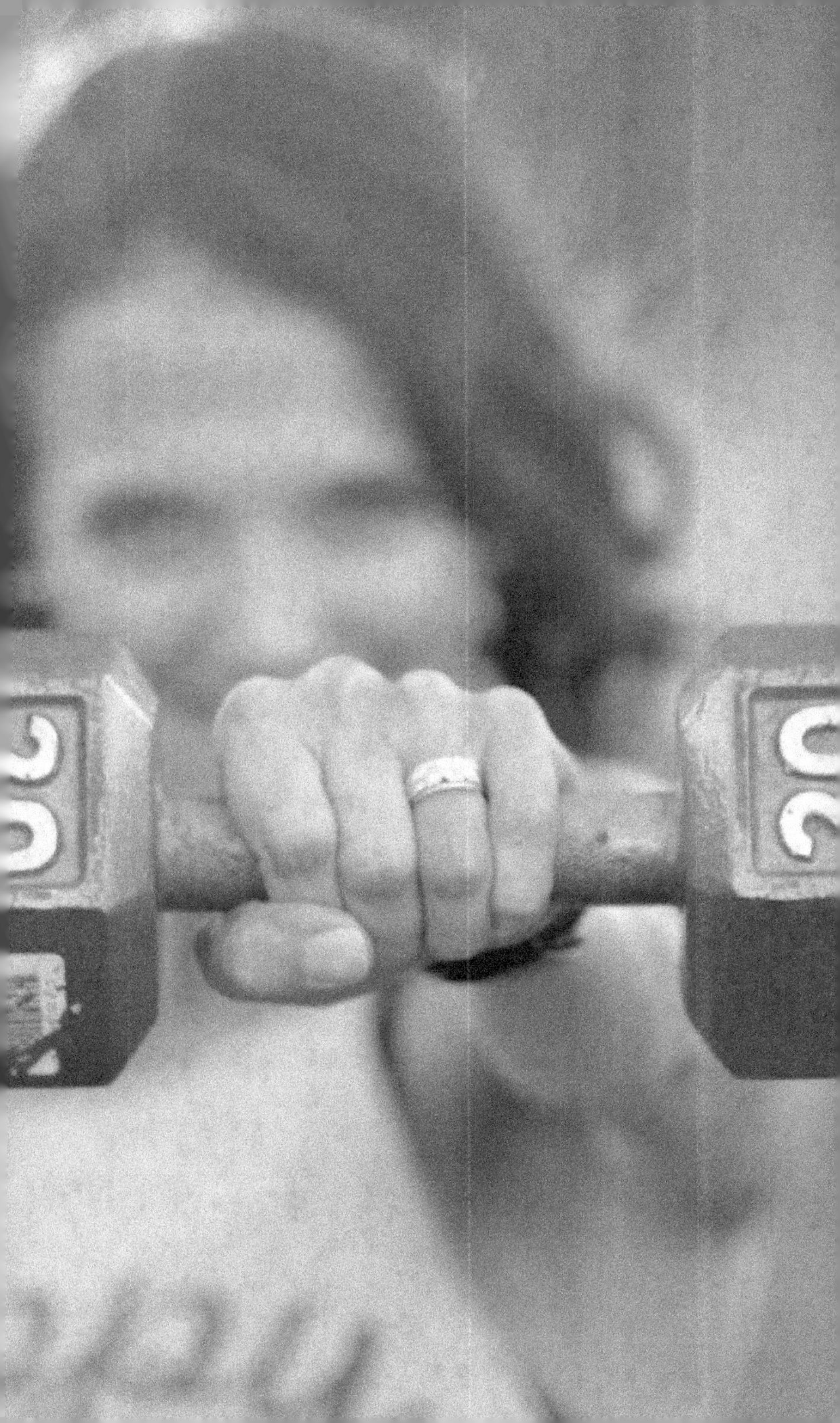

WHAT
TO EXPECT

In this book, you will learn what you need to know in order to create your own custom macros based on your goals. You will also understand what's involved from an exercise and mindset perspective.

I recommend reading through the whole book first, so you have a clear understanding of what's involved in this program.

Then

Go to the "How to Use This Book" section to implement everything you've learned in week-by-week increments. This will ensure you take action in baby steps so you don't get overwhelmed. Many of my clients have lost anywhere from five to 12 pounds over the course of eight weeks by following what you will see outlined.

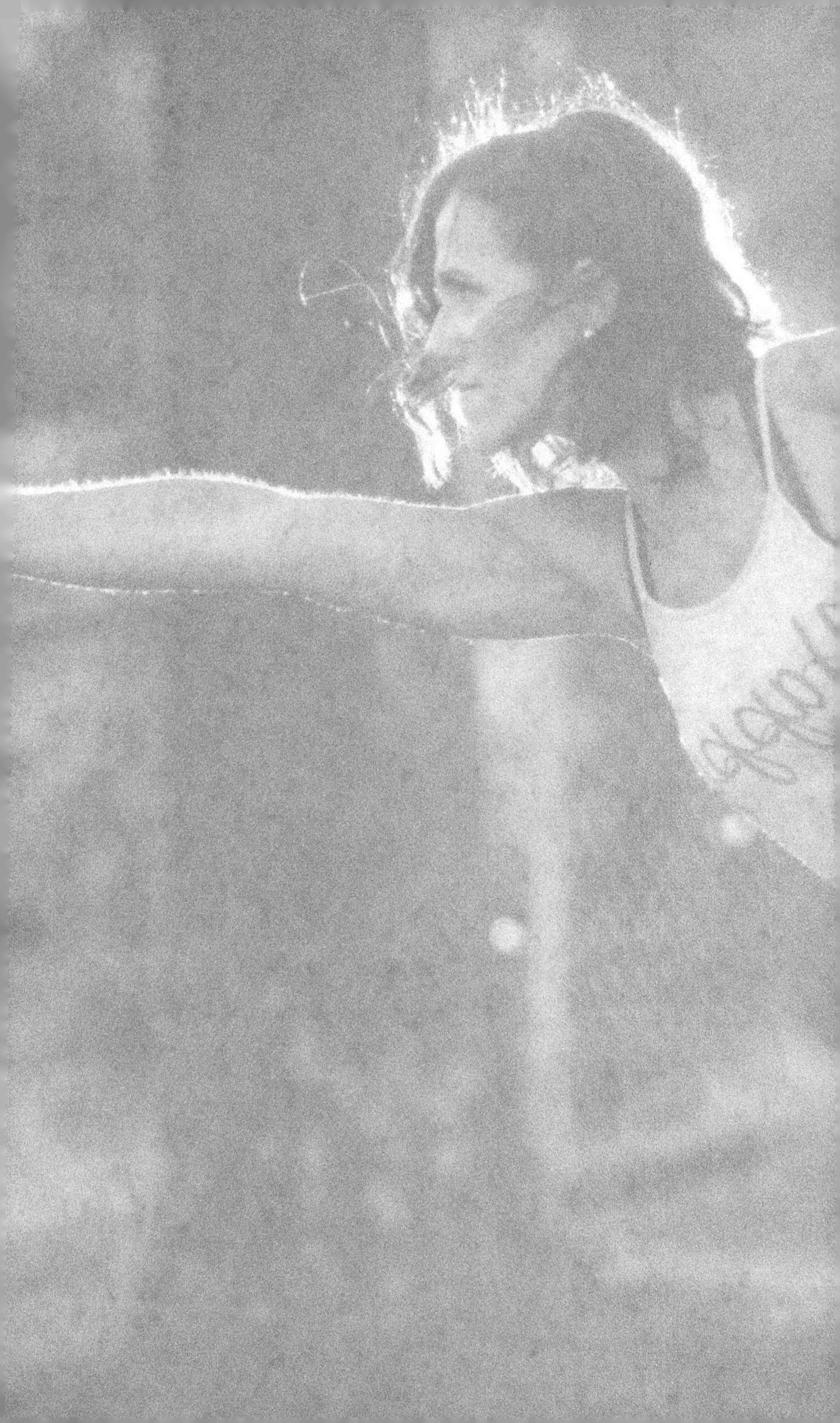

CHAPTER ONE

What Are Macros

MACRO BASICS: Protein, Carbs & Fat

Macronutrients are the building blocks of the foods we eat. It's another way to refer to protein, carbohydrates and fats. Each macro plays a critical role in your diet and how your body functions. Many people believe that managing calories is the most important thing you can do to manage your weight. Your calorie intake does play a huge role in weight loss (calories in versus calories out). However, tracking your macros is even more important when it comes to reaching your goals of losing fat and building muscle (i.e., getting lean).

A great example is if you have a daily calorie goal of 1,500 calories. Essentially, you could eat 1,500 calories of cake or potato chips and reach your goal. However, if you need to eat a certain amount of protein, carbs and fat, you will need to incorporate a more balanced diet to reach that goal. With a more balanced diet comes weight loss as well as a change in your body composition. When you incorporate the right proportions of macronutrients, with a focus on protein and weight training, you can change the composition of your body.

Protein

Protein is made up of a number of amino acids and is essential to building muscle and maintaining your health. Beyond building muscle, protein also plays a role in tissue recovery, hormone production, and cell structure. Plus, eating protein helps to keep you fuller longer because it involves more energy by your body to break it down, giving a slight boost to your metabolism due to this increased effort to digest protein. Carbohydrates and fats can be broken down quicker, which means less effort and less calories used in the digestion process. Protein is the only macronutrient that we cannot store in our bodies. That means if you lack protein in your diet, your body will begin to break down muscle tissue to use as energy. This is why you need to make sure you eat an adequate amount of protein (100g at a minimum).

SOURCES OF PROTEIN:

eggs, chicken, turkey, beef, pork, fish, bison, shellfish, dairy, Greek yogurt, cottage cheese

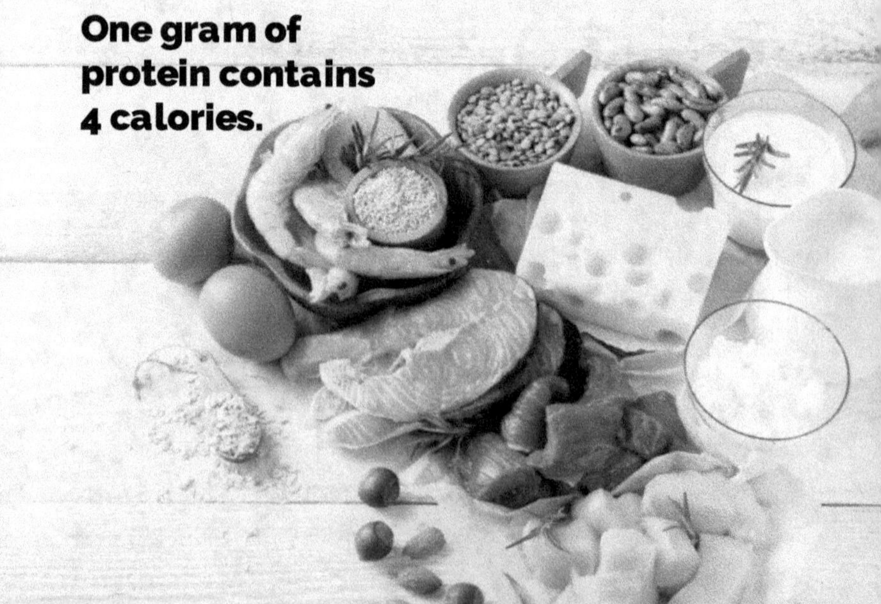

Carbohydrates

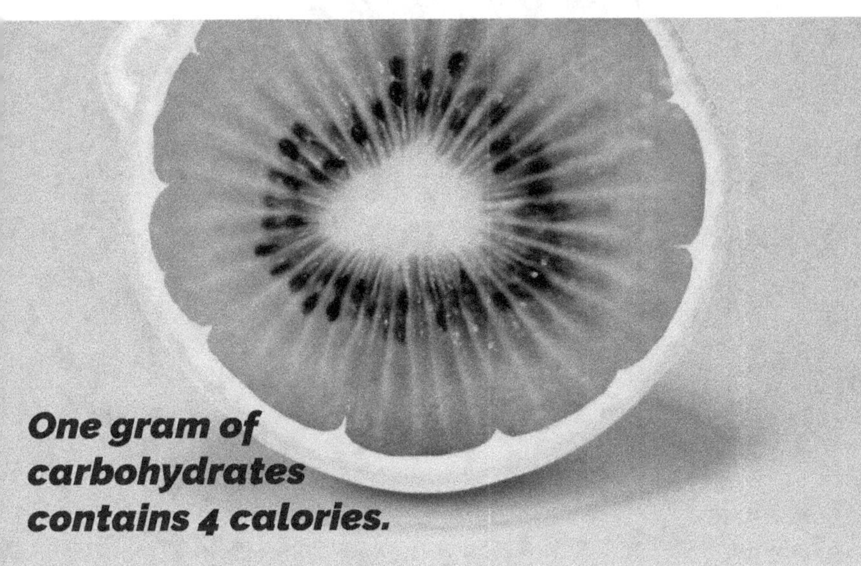

One gram of carbohydrates contains 4 calories.

SOURCES OF COMPLEX CARBS

whole grains, beans, rice, sweet potatoes, kiwi, citrus fruits

SOURCES OF SIMPLE CARBS:

soda, cookies, fruit juice, candy, potato chips, crackers

Carbohydrates are essential for providing your body with energy, and you can find carbs in nearly everything, especially grains, vegetables, fruits and dairy products. This is your body's #1 fuel source. There are two types of carbs: simple and complex. Simple carbohydrates are converted into energy by the body very quickly and can be found in foods such as corn syrup, high-sugar fruits (like pineapple or banana), sugar and fruit juices. Complex carbohydrates are slower to digest and provide more sustained energy. They can be found in foods like whole grains, sweet potatoes, rice and lower-sugar fruits (like apples and berries).

Fats

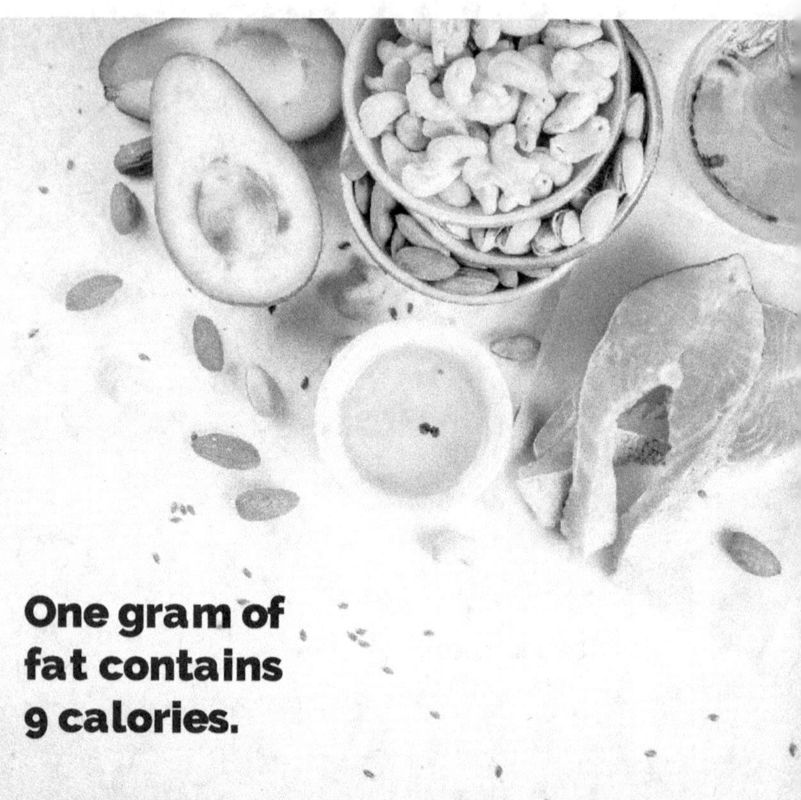

Many people think that if you eat fat, you will get fat. However, fat is vital for the development and overall health of your body. It provides your body with energy, helps transport fat-soluble vitamins, and helps ensure your body functions properly. In addition, you need fat for healthy skin, hair and overall cell function. Healthy fats are easier for the body to break down than less healthy fats, such as fatty red meats, processed lunch meats, margarine, fried foods, etc.

Macros Versus Calories

Many people believe that tracking calories alone will help them to lose weight. And it's true: at the end of the day, weight loss comes down to the calories you consume versus calories that you burn. If you are in a calorie deficit, you will lose weight. If you are in a calorie surplus, you will gain weight.

But let's take a closer look at calories. Macronutrients are what make up food and they translate directly into calories. One gram of protein contains 4 calories, 1 gram of carbohydrates has 4 calories and 1 gram of fat has 9 calories. Tracking calories is important, but tracking calories plus macros is even more important. Why? You could eat 1,500 calories a day and lose weight. But those calories could be French fries and cake-not exactly the best eating plan. Now if you have 1,500 calories and you need to also consume 150 grams of protein, 125 grams of carbohydrates and 45 grams of fat, your diet will look vastly different. In order to hit those macro numbers and stay within your calorie range, you need to be strategic and healthier about your food choices.

Here is what a typical 1,500 calorie day may look like following the macros listed above:

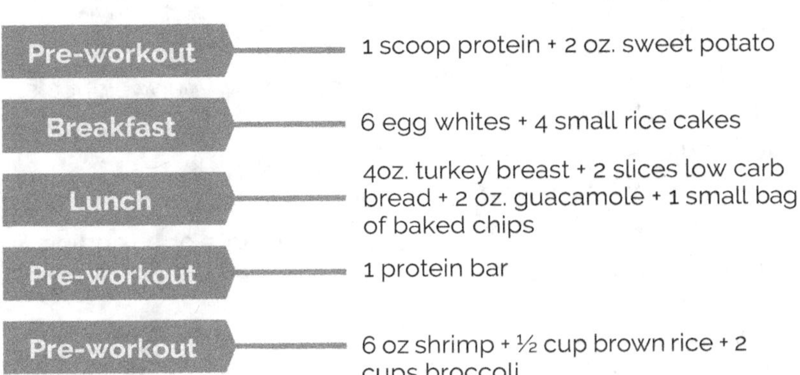

Flexible Dieting

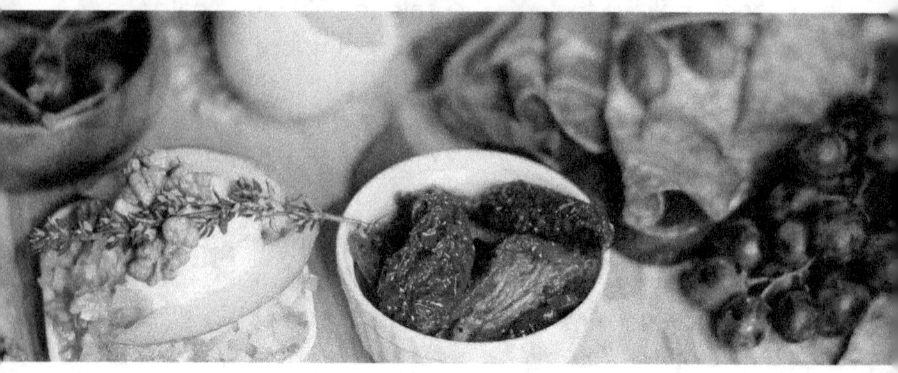

Frequently, macro-tracking is called "flexible dieting" or "If It Fits Your Macros" (IIFYM). It has earned this nickname because nothing is off limits when it comes to your diet. That doesn't mean you can eat cake every day, but it does mean that the diet is flexible enough to incorporate some fun foods and meals on special occasions or when you feel like you need a break.

Rigidity is one of the reasons why diets like Keto or Whole 30 are difficult to sustain over the long term. When you eliminate entire food groups, you feel like you are restricted or deprived. This is what causes binges and it can completely derail an eating plan. Flexible dieting or tracking macros enables you to eat in a sustainable way. And, it can accommodate holidays, special events and times when you feel like you need a little taste of your favorite food. Tracking macros is a lifestyle that you can continue long-term, which makes it a very effective strategy to both lose weight and maintain your weight loss. You will learn more about how to address tricky eating situations, like dining out at restaurants or attending parties, in Chapter 6.

A Note For Women Going Through Menopause

As women get older and go through menopause, hormone changes can impact your weight loss, and many times cause weight gain. As with any diet and exercise program, it's vital to get your doctor's okay and ensure you understand how any medications you may be on could impact your weight loss efforts. In addition, it's crucial to make sure you've had the appropriate testing to understand if you do have a hormonal imbalance or a thyroid condition. Again, these imbalances can hamper your weight loss efforts. If a doctor has cleared you, odds are that you will be able to lose weight during menopause. But, be prepared that it may take a little longer, which can be frustrating. All that said, focusing on a consistent diet with adequate protein and minimal carbs and fat will definitely help you get your weight under control.

Because depending upon your goal – lose fat, gain muscle or lose weight in general - you will need a different proportion of macronutrients. To lose fat or lose weight, you will need less overall calories and macros. You will also want to make sure your diet is

CHAPTER TWO

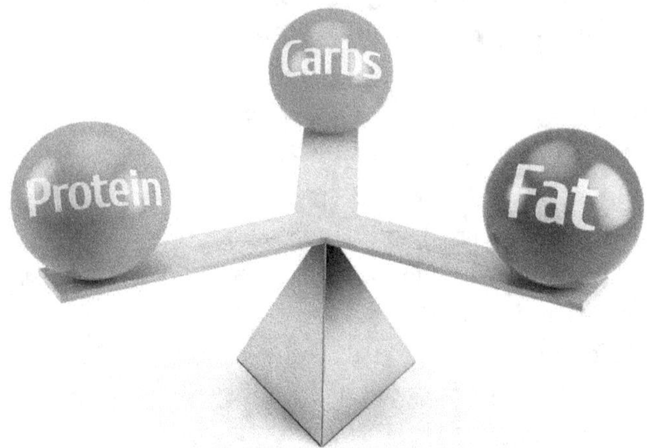

low in fat and moderate in carbohydrates. If you're trying to gain muscle, you will need more calories in terms of more protein and more carbohydrates,

STEP 1

B - **Body**
M- **Mass**
R - **Ratio**

You can find many calculators online for this, like this one:
www.tdeecalculator.net

STEP 2

Calculate your Total Daily Energy Expenditure (TDEE) calories.

You can simply add the calories based on your activity level below.

> **Light:** Any activity that burns an additional 200-400 calories more than your BMR.'

> **Moderate:** Any activity that burns an additional 400-650 calories more than your BMR.

> **Extreme:** Any activity that burns more than about 650 calories more than your BMR.

Depending on your fitness goals, use this guide:

- To lose weight = eat less than TDEE
- To gain weight = eat above TDEE
- To maintain weight = eat at TDEE.

Simple Method for Weight-loss Calories

If you're like me and hate math, the simplest way to determine what your total calorie intake should be to lose weight is to take your current weight and multiply it by 12. For example, a 140-pound woman would consume 1,680 calories to lose weight (140 x 12 = 1,680 calories). Compare this to the example below and you'll see there's only a slight difference in the number of calories she should consume.

STEP 3

Calculate your macros.

Here's a great place to start your breakdown:

1.   **Protein** ratio is set at 1 gram per pound of body weight.
2.   **Fats** are set at 20% of daily energy expenditure.
3.   **Carbohydrate** grams come from the remainder of calories

Here are the calorie values for each micronutrient:

- **1g protein = 4 Calories**
- **1gCarbohydrate = 4 Calories**
- **1g Fat = 9 Calories**

STEP 4

Put it all together!

BMR = 1,437 calories
1,437 + 500 = 1937 (TDEE)
1,937 – 20% = 1,550

Her goal is weight loss (eating under TDEE), so she chooses to eat 1,550 calories. This is 20% less than TDEE, which is a good starting point

Total Calories = 1550,
Macros: Protein 154g | Carbs 156g | Fat 34g come from the remainder of calories

Protein = 154 pounds x 1g = 154g x 4g = 616 calories
Fat = 20% (1550) = 310 calories/9g = 34g = 310 calories
Carb = 624 calories left/4g = 156g

Example: A 40-year-old woman who is 5'4" and 154 pounds and burns an average of 500 calories daily through activity.

Now Let's Figure Out Your Macros

BMR =______________
(visit www.tdeecalculator.net)

TDEE = _____________

_______ (TDEE) - 20% = ______________

PROTEIN = _____ (goal weight) x 1g = ________g X 4 =
__________calories

Fat = 20% X _________(TDEE) = _________ calories/4g =
______g =__________ calories

_________(protein calories) + __________ (carb
calories) = ____________________ (TDEE) =
___________carb calories left

Carbs = ___________(calories left)/4g = ____________g

Total Calories = ___________
Protein = ________________g
Carbs = ________________ g
Fat =_________________g

Meal plan

Here is a sample of three meals based on the macros above. You can eat any combination of meals and snacks to reach your macro goals

Breakfast

- 4 egg whites
- ½ cup (uncooked) instant oatmeal, cream of rice, OR grits
- 10 almonds

Macros: 300 calories, 22g protein, 30g carbs, 10g fat

Lunch

- 4 oz skinless, boneless chicken OR turkey, fish
- 3 oz sweet potato, boiled or baked, without skin
- ½ oz walnuts, shelled

Macros: 315 calories, 25g protein, 22g carbs, 15g fat

Dinner

- 4 oz skinless, boneless chicken breast
- ½ cup long-grain brown rice
- 1 cup broccoli or other green vegetable

Macros: 370 calories, 27g protein, 30g carbs, 15g fat

> You will learn more about how to find out the specific macronutrients of foods in the next chapter.

THE Protein Struggle

When you strive to incorporate 40% of your macros as protein, you will quickly realize that this takes a concerted effort. Your protein intake in grams should generally be equal to your goal body weight in pounds. For example, a woman who weighs 140 pounds and wants to lose 10 pounds should target 130 grams of protein each day. Here are some ways you can hit that number:

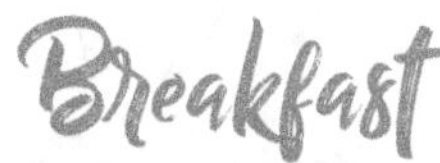

Breakfast

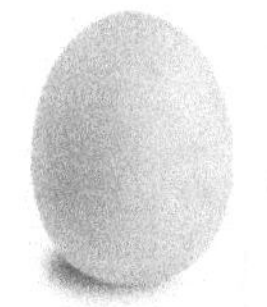

Eat whole eggs or egg whites for breakfast

Lunch

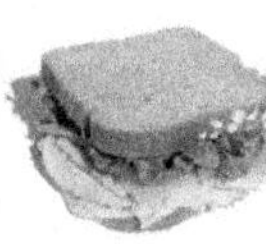

Have a turkey sandwich for lunch

Dinner

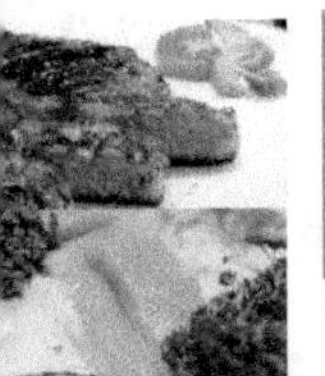

For dinner, have fish or steak

Snacks

For an evening snack, there are numerous options of high-protein ice cream. I personally love Enlightened Birthday Cake popsicles. They're just 70 calories. Other options include Halo, Artic Zero and Pro-Yo.

OTHER

High Protein Options

○ **PROTEIN POWDER** is the fastest, easiest way to reach your quota. I prefer to create protein pudding or protein brownies by mixing in enough water to create a cake-batter-like consistency. This makes a great snack and can be very filling. My favorite protein powders are Beverly International (their graham cracker flavor is amazing) and Quest Protein (so many flavors...all are yummy...my favorites are banana and peanut butter).

○ **BEEF OR TURKEY JERKY** can be easy to find when you are traveling.

○ **CHICKEN** Reasonably priced, versatile and offering countless options, chicken is a no-brainer for protein. You can choose from canned chicken, deli sliced, and plain old chicken breast. Chicken is definitely a staple of my diet.

○ **LOW-FAT OR NON-FAT COTTAGE CHEESE** is a great option that you can mix with fruit.

○ **PLAIN, NONFAT GREEK YOGURT** can be mixed with granola, fresh fruit or powdered peanut butter. Greek yogurt has come a long way and is a great protein addition to your diet.

○ **PROTEIN BARS** are another fast way to eat more protein, but watch the calories and other macros. (I personally like Quest and Power Crunch)

◙ **PROTEIN CHIPS** Quest Protein offers nacho chips and potato chips that are high in protein and quite tasty! In addition, the Rebellion brand offers protein chips in buffalo or BBQ flavor that have amazing macros -- 90 calories per serving and 15g protein!

◙ **HIGH-PROTEIN PEANUT BUTTER** (watch the fat and calories) can be great on rice cakes or on celery

◙ **TOFU**

◙ **BEANS** (watch the carbs)

◙ **QUINOA** (watch the carbs)

◙ **NUTS** (watch the fat)

◙ **SKIM MILK**

◙ **ALMOND MILK** (Unsweetened)

Now you're probably wondering when you get to "eat the foods you love and get lean." Don't worry, I'll be talking more specifically about that in Chapter 6. That said, it's important for you to have a solid understanding of what macros are; which foods contain protein, carbs and fats; how to track those foods; and how to put together healthy meals. This will be very useful when you are traveling, at special events and other scenarios where you are not preparing your own food. You will essentially be able to eyeball the macro breakdown of foods and make good choices, or know how to indulge while not derailing your eating plan.

How to Track Your Macros

Now that you have the basics down pat when it comes to calculating your macros, it's time to learn how to track macros. Tracking is important because it will help guide you in meeting your macro goals, which is key to losing weight and body fat

It will also ensure you eat healthy meals and have a clear understanding of appropriate portions.

In the era of cell phones and apps, there are a variety of macro-tracking options available. One of the most popular and easiest to use is MyFitnessPal. You can download the app for free. There is also a premium version that currently costs $49 per year that lets you customize your macros.

The easiest way to log your food using MyFitnessPal is to do a search or scan the barcode if you're eating packaged food. You will want to double-check that the macros look accurate. Many foods have a green check-market next to them which means they have been verified by others.

You can set your number of meals and snacks in the app, as well as your total number of calories. I do not recommend linking your activity to MyFitnessPal. The reason is because it will add the calories burned, giving you the false belief that you can continue to eat more. In turn, you may end up eating more calories than you need to, which could result in not losing weight and possibly gaining. You can test it out, but generally I like to keep that feature turned off.

HOW TO READ
A Food Label

As a macro counter, you will quickly become very familiar with food labels. These are essentially a road map to what you are eating. The macros are broken down for you on food labels, as well as the calories per serving—all very important information!

If you truly want to understand what you're eating, these little labels are a wealth of information.

Nutrition Facts

Serving size:	..g
Calories:	

% Daily Value*

Total fat	...g	...%
Saturated fat	...g	...%
Cholesterol	...g	...%
Sodium	...g	...%
Total carbohydrate	...g	...%
Dietary Fiber	...g	...%
Sugar	...g	...%
Protein	...g	...%

Vitamin A	...%	Vitamin C	...%
Calcium	...%	Iron	...%

Nutri...

Serving Size 1 egg (50g)

Amount Per Serving	
Calories 70	Calories from
	% Dail
Total Fat 4.5g	
Sat. Fat 1.5g	

STEP 1

Is that giant candy bar one serving or two? Many times, people mistakenly finish an entire bag, bar or drink...only to realize it was 2 or 2.5 servings. That's a diet disaster! To ensure you're consuming the right amount, read the label and measure out a serving either using your hand (see the guide in the Resources section) or a food scale.

STEP 2

If you're tracking macros or following IIFYM, are these fairly equal? Unless the item is rice cakes or beef jerky, you want to ensure any processed food has a fairly equal distribution of macros. This means the calories coming from the different macros are relatively equal. But remember that fat is 9 calories per gram and protein and carbohydrates are 4 calories per gram. Be sure you pay attention to how the calories are divided.

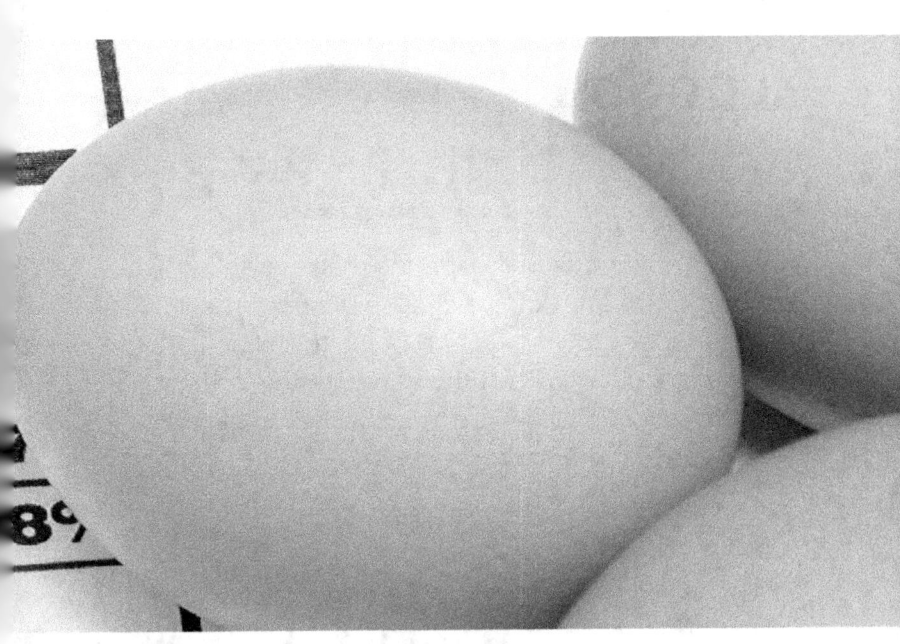

STEP 3

How do these fit into your total allotment for the day? Do they take a big chunk or fit in perfectly?

STEP 4

Can you pronounce all of those ingredients? The more you know and understand, the more you'll make healthier choices. Preservatives, fake sugars and other unknowns are best kept out of your diet to ensure your overall health.

STEP 5

Whenever possible pick items with low fat, low sugar, and low sodium.

ALL GOOD
Things in Moderation

There's nothing more frustrating than struggling with your weight. I know because I've been there. I remember growing up and being told that I was "big-boned" or "healthy." While I knew being healthy should be viewed as a positive, I heard I'm fat, overweight and too healthy.

I love to eat. I love food. When you think about all your daily interactions, most revolve around food. Parties, weddings, work meetings, birthdays...every special occasion has a food component. Not all of the latest 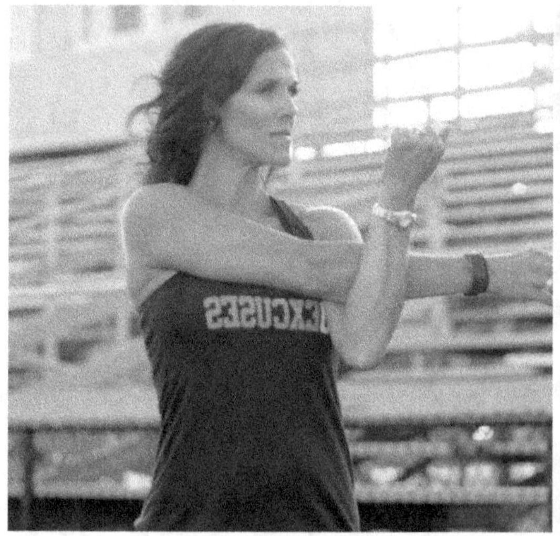 and greatest diets will allow you to enjoy a piece of cake or a glass of wine. For me, that's not living and enjoying life.

When you feel constrained, you want to rebel. Rebelling on your diet means overeating or eating the "wrong" or "bad" foods. News flash: there is no such thing. All food is okay in moderation.

Love pizza? Me too! That means maybe once a month indulging in a slice or two, along with a salad. It does not mean that pizza is for dinner every single Friday night. Variety is the spice of life. That goes for food too! Get creative. Try new recipes. Try revamping or using healthy replacements in an old recipe. You'll be surprised by how much better choices either taste better or how much you can reduce the calories and fat.

Love pasta? Me too! Have you tried spaghetti squash or shirataki noodles? Spaghetti squash is approximately 50 calories per cup, low carb and loaded with fiber. Shirataki noodles are literally 20 calories for an entire bag! They are made from plant fiber and are very versatile, taking on the flavor of whatever you add to them. For example, a little powdered peanut butter and soy sauce creates a nice Thai peanut sauce. Add some vegetables and protein, and you have a low-carb, well-balanced meal!

Love cheese? Me too! Have you ever tried making non-dairy cheese or using Fighter Diet Cheese? These options are lower in fat and calories but give you that cheesy taste – a great option when you're tracking macros.

Love chocolate? Me too! Have you tried making my vegan fudge recipe? (Visit www.allisonjacksonfitness. com and search recipes.) Or, have you tried to make brownies and replace the butter with applesauce or shredded zucchini? Don't knock it until you've tried it! It will help make dessert fit your macros.

There are so many options and resources. Not feeling creative when it comes to healthy cooking or meal prep? Jump on Pinterest or Yummly, or just Google! You will find pages and pages of delicious meals, recipes and ways to eat healthy. You can search "meal prep," "low carb recipe," "healthy dessert," or search by ingredient (e.g., "healthy chicken dinner," "low fat, healthy chocolate dessert").

Before I discovered tracking macros, I was given boring meal plans. Think about eating tilapia, spinach, broccoli, chicken and rice for all of your meals. Sound like fun? Add a wedding, birthday party or work event to the mix, it was sheer torture. Meal plans are incredibly hard to follow when you're thrown into real life and don't want to carry around our food in containers wherever you go. Constantly dragging food everywhere is not convenient – it's stressful!

It's frustrating enough trying to lose weight and watch what you eat. Food is a major part of life. It's how people celebrate, mourn, fuel their bodies, and care for others. That's why having a program that is sustainable and an eating plan that flexes with your life and its ups and downs is so critical to your overall success. That's the beauty of tracking macros!

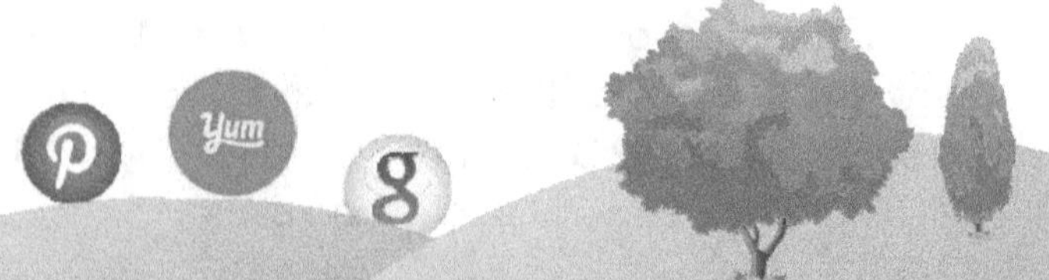

WHAT ABOUT Alcohol

If you enjoy indulging in an alcoholic beverage every now and then, you may be wondering where this fits into your macro plan. Alcohol contains calories and macros. Typically, alcohol is composed of carbs, and you'll want to log alcohol at 7 calories per gram.

That said, you will also want to prioritize your goals. Alcohol inhibits fat loss. It can make you more prone to overeat since it's a depressant, which means your willpower and clarity will be compromised. How often have you randomly eaten food, including chips or other snacks, after consuming one-too-many glasses of wine or beer?

Ideally you should be nearing your weight loss goal before you occasionally indulge in an alcoholic beverage. If having a weekly cocktail is important to you, then you will need to build in additional time to reach your goal.

As a frame of reference, when in competition prep mode, I will refrain from drinking for 12 to 16 weeks. It's not easy, but alcohol also doesn't fit into my goals or priorities. And guess what? A glass of wine and some good dark chocolate taste much better after crushing my goals.

Macro Friendly Meal Prep

Meal prepping doesn't have to be a chore or take all day. When you plan ahead and take some time to outline your meals, you'll find that following an eating plan is much easier and less stressful than ordering takeout!

Meal prepping is important for a variety of reasons. It helps you stick to your grocery budget. It ensures you don't go off track if an unexpected event comes up. Preparing your meals in advance means not running out of certain foods. The list goes on and on. There's a reason why a whole chapter is dedicated to meal prep. I attribute much of my success in competing and maintaining my weight to preparing my meals in advance and tracking my food. If you're serious about losing weight, let's get serious about meal prep. Follow these simple steps and you'll have healthy meals ready to go all week long.

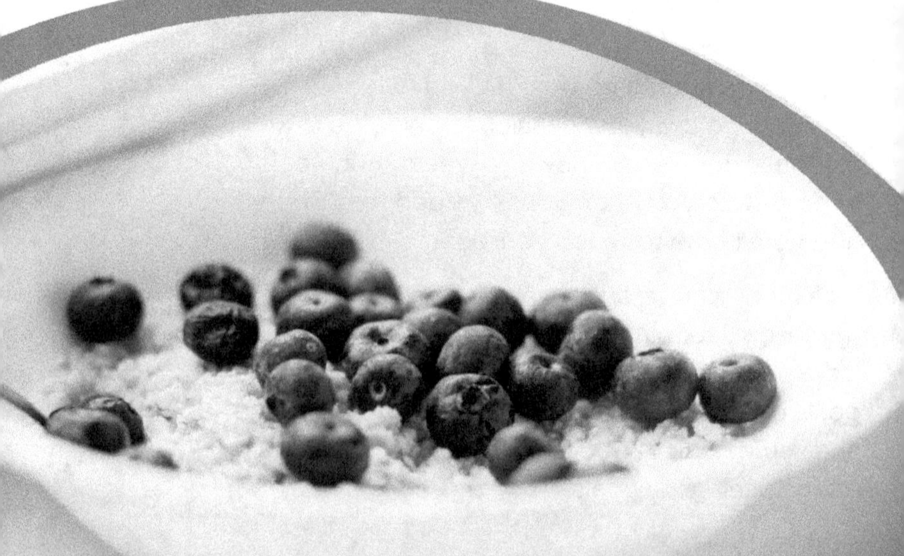

5 SIMPLE STEPS TO MEAL PREP

1 **Look at your weekly grocery store sales flyer and outline your menu for the week.**

I plan all of my meals based on what's on sale. I have several go-to meals that I know my family loves and will also fit into my diet plan. Then, I figure out what to make for breakfast, lunch and dinner each day. It helps to generally eat the same meals each day with some minor changes to keep from getting bored. Minor changes can include switching out different vegetables, such as cauliflower instead of green beans. You can have pork instead of steak or couscous instead of rice. Swapping and substituting provides enormous flexibility. However, you will need to ensure the macros are similar.

Here is a sample of what a typical week looks like for me. I usually keep my meals and snacks the same every day and just alter them each week. It makes prepping and logging much easier.

- Breakfast - 4 egg whites + ½ cup oatmeal
- Lunch - 2 rice cakes, mini guacamole, 4oz turkey
- Snack - Greek yogurt + fresh blueberries
- Dinner - Roasted chicken + 2 cups broccoli + ½ sweet potato

Simple Foods + Similar Meals = Easy Planning

While eating the same thing each day can get boring, you need to think of food as fuel. And, it also helps to get creative with spices and condiments.

For example, Trader Joe's Everything But the Bagel Spice is what I use on my egg whites in the morning to give them some zing. I also live by McCormick Grill Mates Smokehouse Maple Spice for my veggies. It tastes amazing on broccoli, cauliflower and string beans. I even have my 15-year-old son using it.

Other spices and condiments that I've fallen in love with include Trader Joe's Chili Lime, Jalapeno Salt and crystallized lemon and lime (all available on Amazon). The lemon and lime do not include salt (although it may taste like it) and there is a crystallized lime with cilantro and garlic that is amazing as well. If you are watching your salt intake, Mrs. Dash and Flavor God are two brands that offer no-salt or minimal sodium options.

You want to look at the ingredients and also be sure to be conscious of how much you use. Some may be loaded with salt or sugar so be sure to use as little as possible. Most of these spices are so strong, a little goes a long way!

Create shopping list

3

I typically order my groceries online from ShopRite. It's the best $10 I spend for the time and stress that it saves me. I'm able to shop from a list and use coupons, which helps me stay on track, save money and save my precious time and sanity. Your shopping list should include all of the items you will need for all of your meals.
I typically shop online Saturday night and pick up my order Sunday morning or early afternoon.
Then, I spend 60-90 minutes meal prepping once I pick up my order.

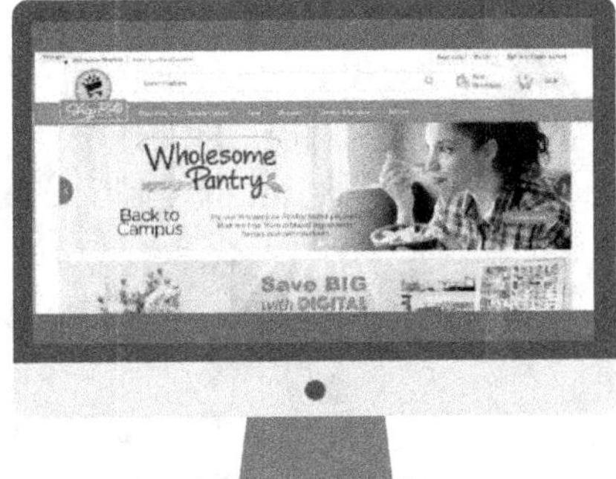

Get out all of your essential prep tools.

4

Once you get your order, dig out all of the tools and gadgets you will need to prepare for the week. This includes a food scale, containers, labels or Post-Its, spices and be sure to clear out some room in the fridge.

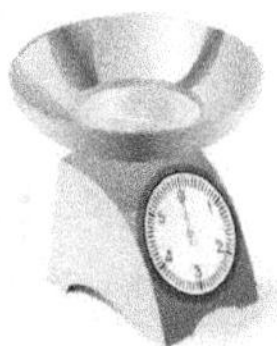

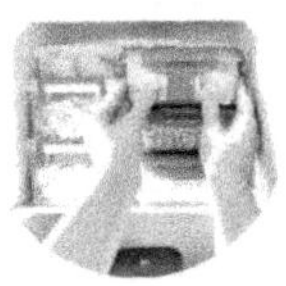

5   **Cook or prep food to be cooked.**

Now you don't necessarily have to cook all of your food ahead of time, but you can if you want to. What I do is prepare all of my meals and keep them refrigerated so I can just pop them in the oven and have dinner ready to go within 30 minutes of walking in the door. For example, Crockpot meals can be put in the Crockpot (or Instant Pot) and then into the fridge for whenever that meal comes up during the week. I like to buy frozen bags of veggies that can easily be microwaved at home for dinner, or at work if I include them for lunch. It's easy to roast large quantities of chicken, vegetables and potatoes. But you can also just have them ready to go into the oven. For example, another one of my staple meals is sheet pan chicken fajitas. I slice up the chicken, peppers and onions, coat them in fajita mix and put them on a sheet pan. Then, I cover the pan and leave it in the fridge until that meal is needed.

While meal prep may take some time at first, once you get the hang of it, it becomes second nature and just another part of your routine.

MEAL

Prep Tools

When it comes to meal prep, there are few things to keep in mind. First, you need to gather all the tools you'll need. Then, you'll need to plot out exactly what meals you're going to make for the week. The way I typically do this is:

1. I will look at the grocery store flyer to see what's on sale.

2. From there, I'll outline what the week looks like by looking at my family's calendar. I'll plan for events on the schedule like sports meetings or other evening activities.

3. For days when my family does have activities on the calendar, I'll make sure dinner is planned for those evenings are quick and easy.

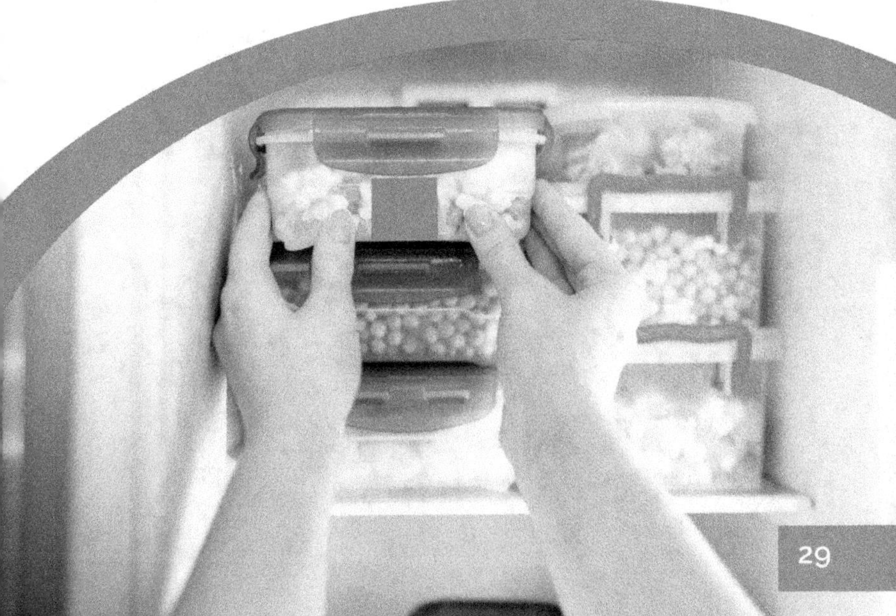

When you fail to plan, you plan to fail. Following a proper diet accounts for 90% of your results, but it can be easy to have your diet derailed. That's why preparing meals ahead of time is so important! Here are the tools you need to get started:

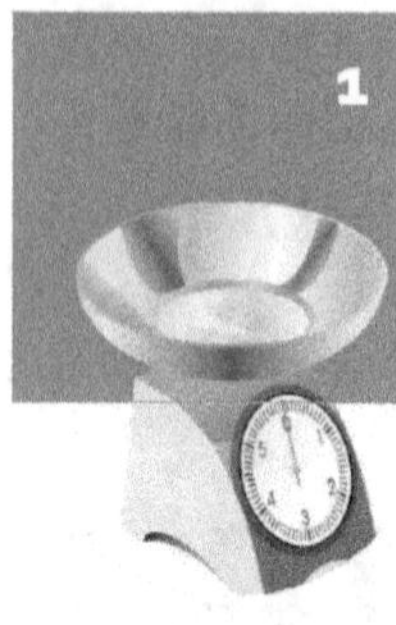

Food Scale – Portion control is easy when you can physically measure your food

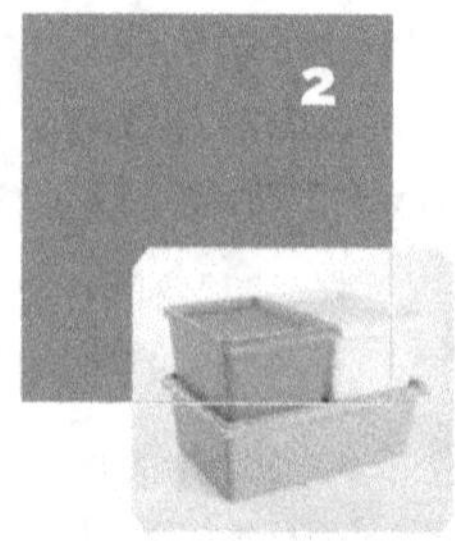

Containers – Grab-and-go containers make storage easy, whether in the fridge or in your lunch bag

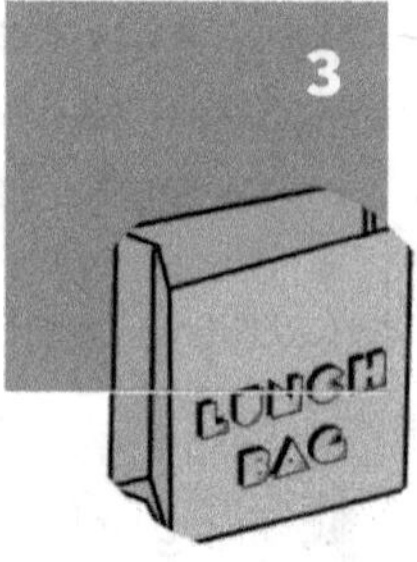

Lunch bag – Not only will you save money packing your lunch, you'll know exactly what you're eating and how it was prepared.

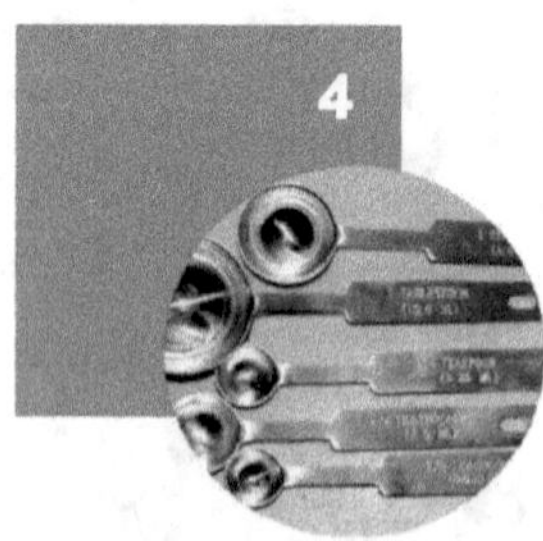

Measuring spoons – helpful for measuring spices and other smaller quantities

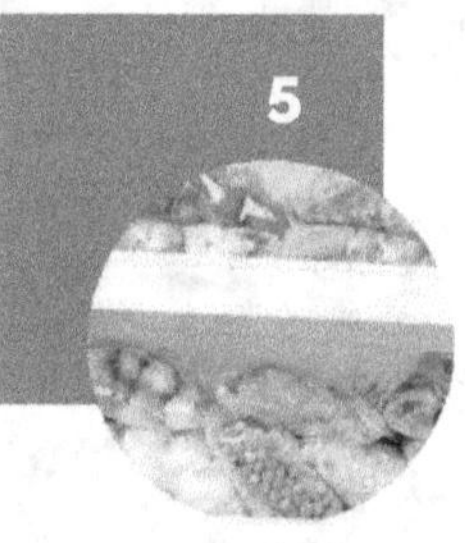

Storage bags – multiple sizes for those items that don't need a container, like nuts or dried fruit

PLANNING YOUR

Menu for the Week

Now let's look at how you should plan your menu for the week. Typically, families have lots of activities and sports going on, which can do real damage to your best-laid plans for dinner. Dinner is my main focus, but I do also like to plan ahead for lunch and breakfast. My family typically eats the same things for these meals, just maybe a different cereal, or one day they'll have frozen pancakes or waffles.

Look at Your Social Calendar

The first thing you should do is take a look at your social calendar. I like to keep a desk calendar on our counter where everyone in my family puts all of our social activities, events and meetings. Another option is to have your calendar online, using a service such as Google Calendar. This enables everyone to log on and know what's going on when. However, I like to have the dinner meal plan written out and posted on the refrigerator.

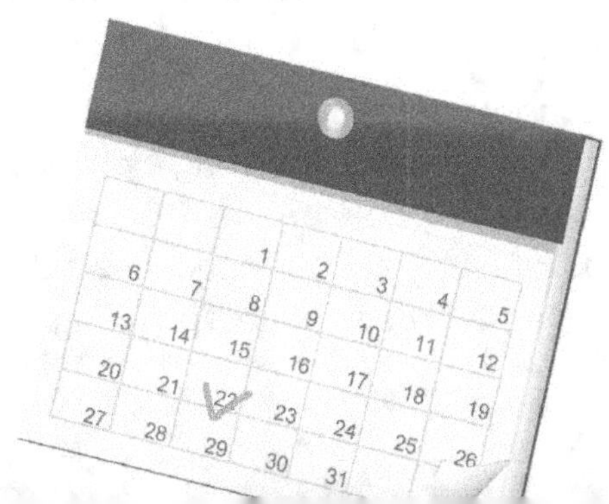

Regardless of your kids' ages or how many family members do you have, it's good to get your family involved in your planning. There's nothing worse than having meals that your family does not enjoy. I know I, for one, go crazy when my kids don't like a meal that I make a concerted effort to create. There are a few ways to get your family involved. They can help you with the online grocery shopping, or they can help you come up with the recipes and meals for breakfast, lunch or dinner. For example, I like to let my 12-year- old daughter pick some of the dinners that we will have. Another option is to get your kids involved in the cooking, depending on how old they are. Here are some examples for different age ranges:

- **Pre-school/ toddlers** – At this age, you can begin getting them used to understanding the tools used in cooking. They can gather all of the tools and foods that you need to start food prepping.

- **Elementary school age** – Kids at this age can help with stirring or mixing foods, putting food into bowls or pans, and reading through the steps of the recipe.

- **Middle school age** – Depending upon how much kitchen experience they have, you can enlist their help with chopping, making a salad, and putting cooking food into containers.

- **High school age** – Hopefully your children are well versed in food prep and cooking. You may be able to outsource the whole process to them! When your family has a vested interest in the meals they eat, it can make family time and meal planning much more enjoyable.

I always say that the mind is a sieve. So, when it comes to meal planning, make sure to write it down. I like to post our weekly meal plan on a refrigerator so everyone can see. This also helps when people come home before you so they can get started on dinner. The first one home starts the process. This could be setting the table or getting the food ready to be cooked. Again, how you cook your meals all depends on your time schedule, what time you get home and what time your family gets home. It's important to be flexible and to have an open mind when it comes to meal planning. Nothing is perfect and there will be times when you question why you made a certain meal because it took so much effort, was too complicated or didn't turn out so great. I find that Crockpot meals and one-pan meals are the best for during the week. I would save any elaborate new recipes for over the weekend when you have more time and energy.

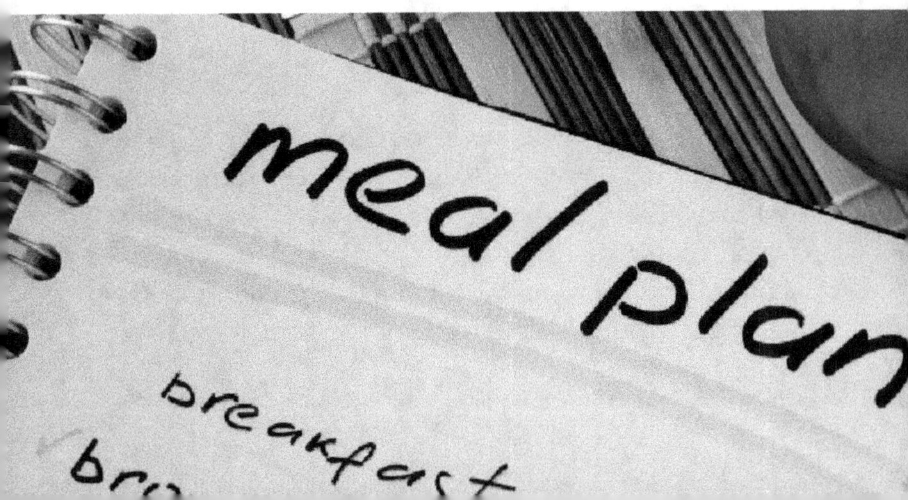

How to Strategically Grocery Shop

To get started with your meal prep, the first thing you're going to need to do is go grocery shopping. Here are some tips on how I approach grocery shopping in order to save money as well as stick to my eating plan.

Buy What's On Sale

First, you want to get the grocery sales flyer. Then, you want to see what's currently on sale. What's on sale is going to determine what you have for breakfast, lunch and dinner that week. Typically, I buy the same things, but try to buy in bulk when those items are on sale. For example, I will buy chicken breast, frozen vegetables, pasta sauce, and anything else that is on sale that I can stock up on.

Typically, the items that are on sale are on the cover of the flyer. It's easy to see what you should buy based on looking at the front and the back. Usually the meats that are on sale around the front, and the vegetables

Use Coupons

When it comes to coupons, I don't go crazy using them. However, I will use them for things that we buy regularly. I will also use coupons for things we may want to try. I have a coupon book that keeps them organized, and I try to review them as I put my shopping list together. Cutting coupons takes a lot of time, so this might not be something that

you will want to do or need to do. It's completely up to
you and your preference. But, if saving money is a goal,
coupons are a huge help.

Order Online for Pick Up or Delivery

When it comes to grocery shopping, there are so many
options available, from ordering online to immediate
delivery to picking up your groceries. There are numerous
ways to save money and time. The beauty of having your
groceries picked up or delivered is you can order them
online and then schedule the pickup or delivery time.

Personally, I like to order my groceries online and then
pick them up. But I'm a control freak and I do like to see
what I am getting. However, I will sometimes have them
delivered. It depends how much food I am ordering. This
saves a huge amount of time and effort for you to go to
the grocery store, find everything, check out, bag your
groceries, and drive home. It's definitely money well spent.

Order the Same Thing Each Week

When you begin to order your groceries online, you will
quickly notice that you ordered the same things every
week. If your grocery store saves your shopping list (which
most typically do), you can just check off the items that
you need to buy, making shopping much faster and
simpler. Matching of coupons is also much easier if you
buy the same things each week. Along the same lines,
I also keep a running list of items we run out of on the
refrigerator. I grab my list before I log online to order my
groceries to ensure that I get everything that we need.

HOW TO MEAL PREP
When You Didn't Grocery Shop

Life can sometimes (okay, many times) get in the way of your best-laid plans. For example, last month sports and a wedding derailed my normal grocery shopping and food prep game plan. What's a girl to do? I raided the freezer and pantry to see what I could make for the week. Then, I figured out when I could hit the grocery store for those must-have items (i.e., milk, eggs, etc.).

I also try to keep at least 2-3 meats (bought in bulk on sale, of course) in the freezer for these kinds of emergencies. I typically will get pork (tenderloin, chops), steak (flank, sirloin, T-bone), chicken (breast, skinless thighs), lean ground beef, turkey or chicken (95%/5% for beef and 93% or 99% for poultry) and ham steaks.

Here is typically how a week from the freezer may look

- Sheet-pan chicken fajitas
- Grilled bone-in pork chops
- Steak
- Pasta (for the husband and kids -- leftover protein-based meal for me)
- Leftover night
- Tacos
- Breakfast for dinner (egg white veggie omelet for me and bacon and egg on a bagel for the family)

Usually we have leftovers, so you could have a dinner of leftovers, buffet-style, or bring those to lunch with you.

Now that you have your tools in check, let's get started on some easy meal-prep recipes.

Sheet-Pan Chicken Fajitas

INGREDIENTS:

2 lbs. chicken breast
3 bell peppers
1 onion
Fajita mix (or make your own)

1. Line a sheet pan with aluminum foil.
2. Spray with oil.
3. Slice up everything and spread it over the sheet pan in an even layer
4. Sprinkle fajita seasoning over everything.
5. Bake at 400°F for 20-25 min.
6. Eat over greens,

Makes approx. 8 servings.

1 serving = 4 oz. chicken + ½ cup onions and peppers

Macros: 160 calories, 21g protein, 4g carbs, 6g fat

Crockpot Teriyaki Chicken

INGREDIENTS:

12 boneless, skinless chicken
thighs (I always throw in a chicken
breast or two for myself)
1/4 cup honey
3/4 cup low-sodium soy sauce
6 tbsps. cider vinegar
3/4 tsp ground ginger
3/4 tsp minced garlic
1 tsp pepper

1. Place chicken in crockpot.
2. In a large bowl, combine remaining ingredients.
3. Pour over chicken.
4. Cover and cook on low for 6 hours or until chicken is tender.
5. Serve over rice. I also like to include some broccoli.

Makes approx. 8 servings.

1 serving = 4 oz. chicken breast

Macros: 140 calories, 21g protein, 0g carbs, 6g fat

Ground Beef + Cabbage Stir Fry

(aka Crack Slaw)

INGREDIENTS:

1 lb. ground extra lean beef or 99%
fat free ground chicken or turkey
1 red onion
1 small bag broccoli slaw or coleslaw

1. Spray a large frying pan with oil.
2. Brown ground meat in frying pan.
3. Add onions, cook until translucent..
4. Add in coleslaw. Mix thoroughly.
5. Season as you'd like.
6. Cover and cook 15-20 min. until cabbage is wilted.

Makes approx. 5 servings.

1 serving = 5 oz.

Macros: 140 calories, 21g protein, 0g carbs, 6g fat

CHAPTER FIVE

While nutrition makes up approximately 90% of your overall results, including focused workouts will help fast track your results.

Working out is important not only for heart health, but also for your joints, bones, tendons and muscles. From flexibility to reflexes, exercise will help ensure you remain agile and physically healthy. Many of my clients have not only lost weight when they incorporate short, effective workouts, they also have more energy, sleep better and clarity and overall confidence. Working out will also increase your motivation. I had one client go from not exercising for years, to running a 5k!

Why You Need Weight Training

Whether your goal is to gain muscle, lose fat, remain injury-free or just maintain a healthy lifestyle, weight training will get you there. It can help you enjoy the activities you love, and it doesn't take a lot of time to incorporate it into your exercise routine.

Here's why

1. **Lean tissue, including skeletal muscle developed during exercise, takes much more energy to maintain than fat.**

That means the more muscle you have, the more calories you burn, even when you're not working out. That means you will event-ually be able to eat more without gaining weight. Obviously having lean muscle will lead to overall weight loss and the ability to maintain that weight loss. Now are you ready to incorporate weight training into your routine? This boost in your metabolic rate makes weight training the perfect complement to your cardio or yoga training, which is sometimes associated with a slower of metabolic rate.

2 **Weight training is the fountain of youth. It stops muscle loss in its tracks.**

Do you want to be that elderly, frail person who has trouble climbing stairs or walking? Skeletal muscle atrophy increases sharply for sedentary individuals over 50, leading to a higher injury risk and even chronic disease risk. As we age, muscle mass declines around 0.18 kg per year. The good news is that this can be completely reversed with weight training.

3 **Build better bones with weight training.**

Lifting weights is the single best way to improve and maintain bone density. A 1999 review in Medicine & Science in Sports & Exercise led by Jean Mayer found that resistance training increased bone density and improved other risk factors better than pharmacological and nutritional approaches.

Stronger bones will provide your body with better support and you will be better able to resist breaking upon impact. And, your stronger legs and core will be more stable and resilient as you move through the world, preventing stumbles, missteps and falls.

④ Protect and build resistance in your joints.

Weight training will improve the strength and stability of all the joints in your body. Regardless of your age, anyone can get injured, even if you're just walking down the street. Plus, anyone engaging in strenuous sports or physical activity like running, biking, Cross Fit or other intense workouts increases their risk of injury while training.

But strength training is the best defense against injury. Stronger muscles will support your joints better. That means there will be less of a chance of blowing out your knee or hyper-extending your elbow. You will also be less likely to strain or sprain a joint.

With all of these benefits, it's easy to see why resistance training can do a lot to keep you pain-free.

What's not to love about strength training? It can make you stronger, healthier and less injury-prone.

EFFECTIVE Workout Plans

You do not have to spend hours in the gym working out to get the body of your dreams. Even when I'm in the midst of preparing for figure competitions, I spend no more than an hour in the gym.

Whether you work out at home or a gym, you can get in an effective workout with as little as 10-15 minutes. If you have more time and you're feeling ambitious, shoot for 20-30 minutes 3-5 times per week. Ideally, you would do weight training or body weight workouts (either at home or at the gym) 3 times a week on Mondays, Wednesdays and Fridays, do two cardio sessions on Tuesdays and Thursdays and then one enjoyable physical activity on Saturday (e.g., golf, yoga, hiking, etc.). Sunday would be a total rest day.

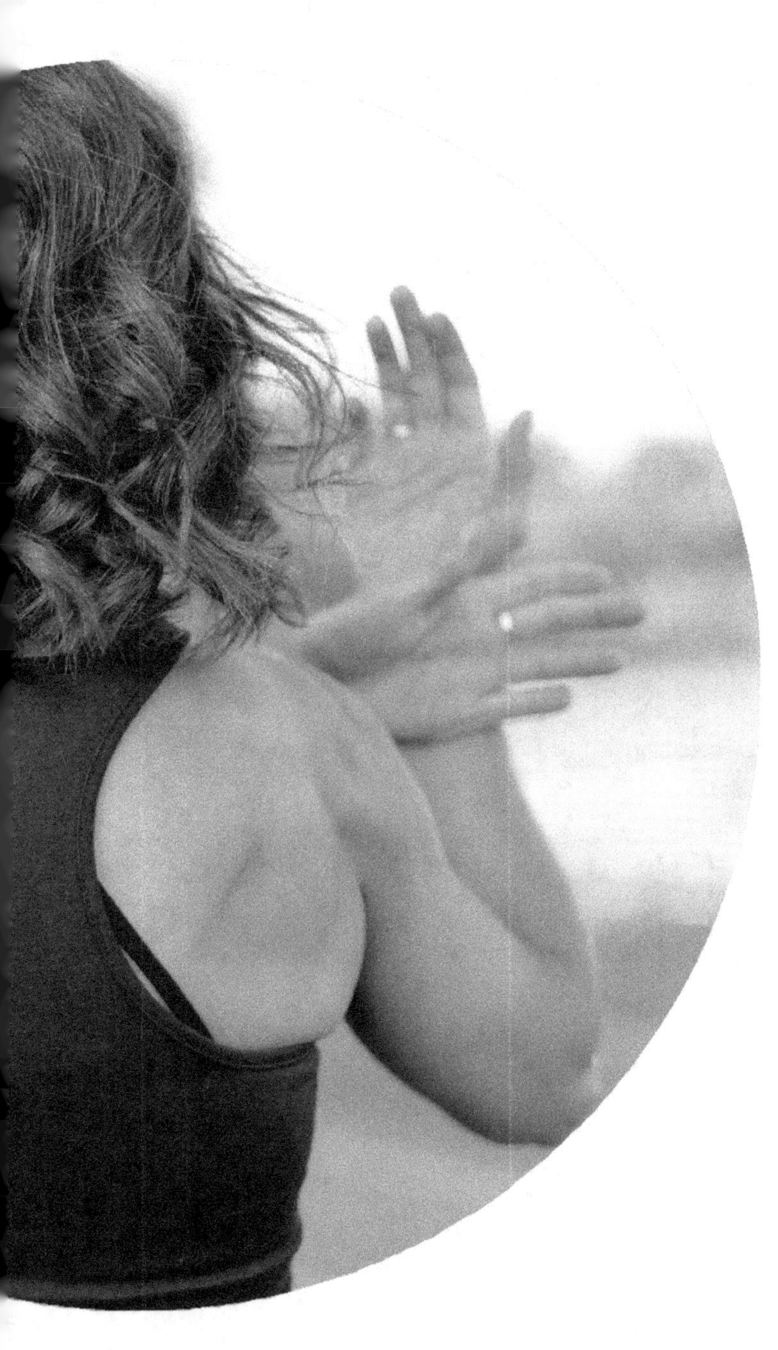

Home Workout (20-30 min)

Complete this workout 3 times per week, preferably on Monday, Wednesday and Friday.

You will need dumbbells (depending upon your strength, start at five pounds) or resistance bands (low to medium strength for beginners).

- Push-ups
- Dumbbell military press
- Dumbbell lateral raise
- Alternating dumbbell curl
- Dumbbell overhead extension
- Single bent dumbbell row
- Squats
- Deadlift with dumbbell
- Walking lunges
- Dumbbell lateral raise
- Standing calf raise
- Crunch

Do 3 sets 10-12 reps for each exercise.

Visit www.allisonjacksonfitness.com/flab-to-fab for a video outlining how to do these exercises.

Gym Workout (20-30 min)

Complete this workout 3 times per week, preferably on Monday, Wednesday and Friday.

- Bench press
- Chest fly machine
- Shoulder press machine
- Dumbbell lateral raise
- Cable EZ bar bicep curl
- Dumbbell overhead extension
- Wide lateral pulldown (cable machine)
- Seated row (cable machine)
- Leg press
- Leg extension
- Leg curl
- Calf raise machine
- Ab machine

Do 3 sets 10-12 reps for each exercise.

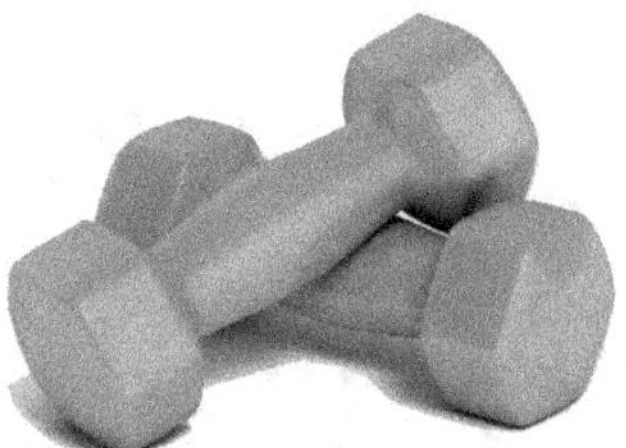

Cardio

You have several options here. One cardio session can be any of the following:

> 30 min. steady-state (breathing heavy—on a scale of 1-10, difficulty = 5 or 6)

> 20 min. HIIT (high-intensity interval training)

THE BEST Exercise

Everyone wants that magic bullet. What is the #1 exercise to get results? Well, first, it's the exercise that you will do and enjoy. It could be yoga, weight training, running, cycling or any other movement. But, to truly change your body, you must include weight training. Lifting weights makes your muscles and bones stronger. It gives you that toned look that everyone strives for.

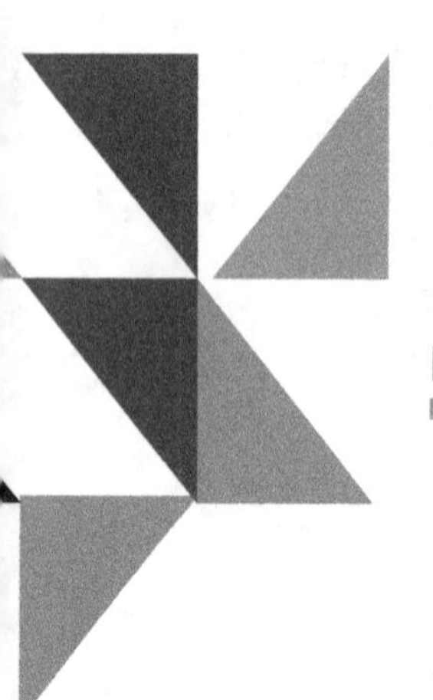

And, building muscle is not easy. You need to lift heavy, and by heavy, I mean you should struggle a little bit and get outside of your comfort zone.

NEAT

What if I told you that fidgeting and moving around throughout the day could aid your weight loss efforts? Well, it's true. When you burn these calories, it's called NEAT (non-exercise activity thermogenesis). This non-exercise-related calorie burn also include sleeping, eating, standing, and fidgeting. Depending upon how much you move throughout the day, whether you have a desk job versus being a waitress, you could burn 100 calories per hour or 200 calories per hour. (This depends upon your weight, how much you move, etc.)

Knowing that, your goal is to get in as much movement as you can throughout the day, because extra activity could be equal to a formal workout. What are some ways to get in extra **NEAT**?

- Stand more, or get a standing desk at work if you have a desk job.
- Wash your car by hand.
- Pace the sidelines at your kids' athletic games.
- Take some extra laps around the grocery store when you're shopping.
- Walk briskly through the mall and take the long route, including the stairs.
- Take the long way to the water cooler or bathroom at the office.
- Walk to a co-worker's desk instead of emailing or calling them.
- While you're on the phone, pace around if possible.
- Make meetings walking meetings whenever you can.
- Take the stairs instead of the elevator.
- Don't use the drive-thru; park far away and walk inside.

Throughout your day, find ways to get more steps in. Get a step counter or use your smartphone to track how far you walk each day. Make it a game. If you start at 5,000, shoot for 7,000, then 10,000 steps each day. As little as 100 extra calories burned each day translates to approximately 10 lbs. lost in a year; 200 calories are equal to a 20-pound loss—and that's without even breaking a sweat!

CHAPTER SIX

Afraid of going to a restaurant or party because you're on a diet? If you've experienced this before, you can let that fear go. When you track your macros, you have complete flexibility and freedom to make choices based on your macro number. That means no food is off limits. This chapter is going to help you understand how to take back control and feel confident during those special occasion situations, whether it's a wedding, party or work event.

Eating Out? Strategies for Healthy Restaurant Options

One of the quickest ways to derail your diet is to eat out. It's difficult to know how much oil, butter or other ingredients are used when a chef prepared your meal. Does that mean you can never eat out again? Hells no! But you do need to take some precautions and properly planning to ensure you keep your eating on track. Here are five simple tips to help

1 Look at the menu before you get to restaurant.

How many times have you gone out to eat with friends and started chatting before being able to thoroughly review the menu? Then, you're left scrambling to order when the waiter shows up. The best way to keep that from happening is to go online and see if the restaurant has their menu posted (most do). Quickly scan the menu to ensure you have healthy options or so you can begin to strategize .how you can customize your order.

2 **Choose grilled, steamed, baked or braised.**

When selecting lean protein (which should be a good portion of your meal), opt for grilled, steamed, baked or braised. These options typically don't use a ton of oil, unlike deep frying or pan frying. For extra credit, ask for minimal butter and oil during the cooking process.

3 **Stay away from sauces, oil and butter.**

Since you don't know how much is being used, ask for any special sauces or creams on the side. This way you can determine how much sauce you use (if you use any at all). This helps you to gauge how much you put on and take better control of the meals you eat at restaurants.

4 **Desperate times call for desperate measures.**

Stuck going to a restaurant like Five Guys where you have extremely limited options? Choose wisely by having a burger wrapped in lettuce with lots of veggies and no sauces. When in doubt, choose a lean protein and veggies. Nearly every restaurant has a salad with grilled chicken as an option. And when that isn't an option, you will need to get creative and improvise.

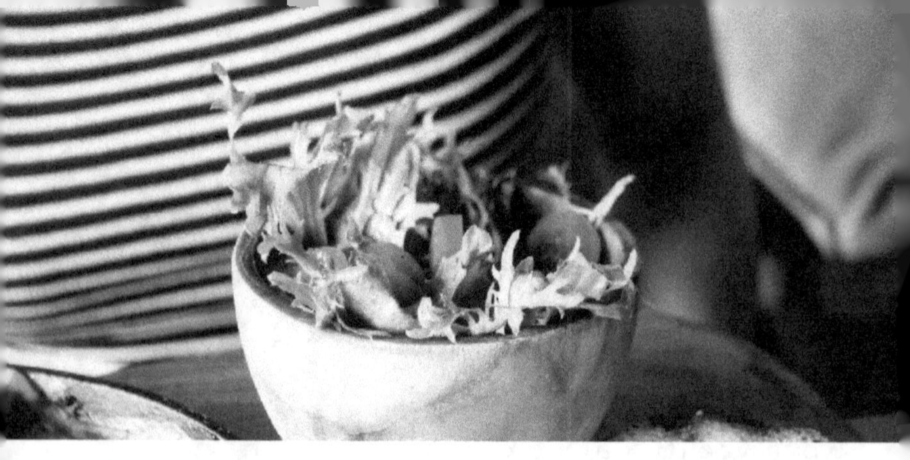

5 Pick healthy restaurants when possible.

If the restaurant choice is up to you, select an establishment where you know you can get some healthy options. For example, we have a local diner that has so many options, from egg white omelets to salads to grilled chicken dishes. Other fast food places that have diet-friendly menus include Chipotle, Panera, Chili's and Starbucks. Even McDonald's, Burger King and Wendy's have decent salad selections.

Ready to Indulge?

Here's how

Understandably, there will be times when you want to indulge. For me, I love enjoying a special meal for my birthday or wedding anniversary. You can definitely have a meal of your choice and enjoy it without any guilt. How? Eat a little bit less throughout the day and drink lots of water.

For your special meal, don't eat like the ship is going down. Make selections that you thoroughly enjoy and relish. Have a glass of wine, enjoy dessert and make the meal a true experience. Don't scroll on your phone as you mindlessly eat. Afterwards, go back to your eating plan. One meal will not completely erase your efforts. However, if this becomes part of your regular routine, it definitely will hamper reaching your goals. Try to follow the 80-20 rule. Eat healthy and in moderation 80% of the time and then you can enjoy a treat 20% of the time.

Again, this is if your goal is to lose weight. If you're just trying to maintain your goal. Your strategy will be a little different and you may be able to have this type of meal every week or every two weeks.

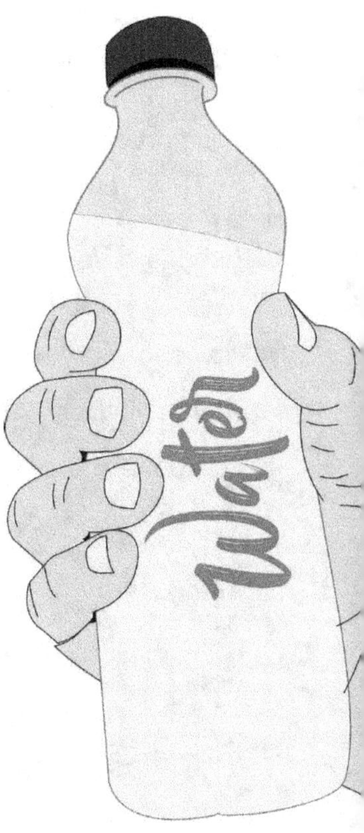

Ways to Celebrate Food-Focused Holidays - That Don't Involve Food

When you think about most of the holidays celebrated in the U.S. – Thanksgiving, July 4th, Christmas, Easter, Hanukah – they all revolve around food. Is it possible to celebrate without wrecking your diet? Of course, there is! While food may be a large part of the equation, here are some suggestions for other activities to include during your celebration that can help reduce the focus on food. I know when I attend holiday gatherings or special occasions, it can be difficult to not mindlessly eat the entire time.

- Play some board games with the family.

- Share your best or funniest family memories.

- Take a walk after your meal.

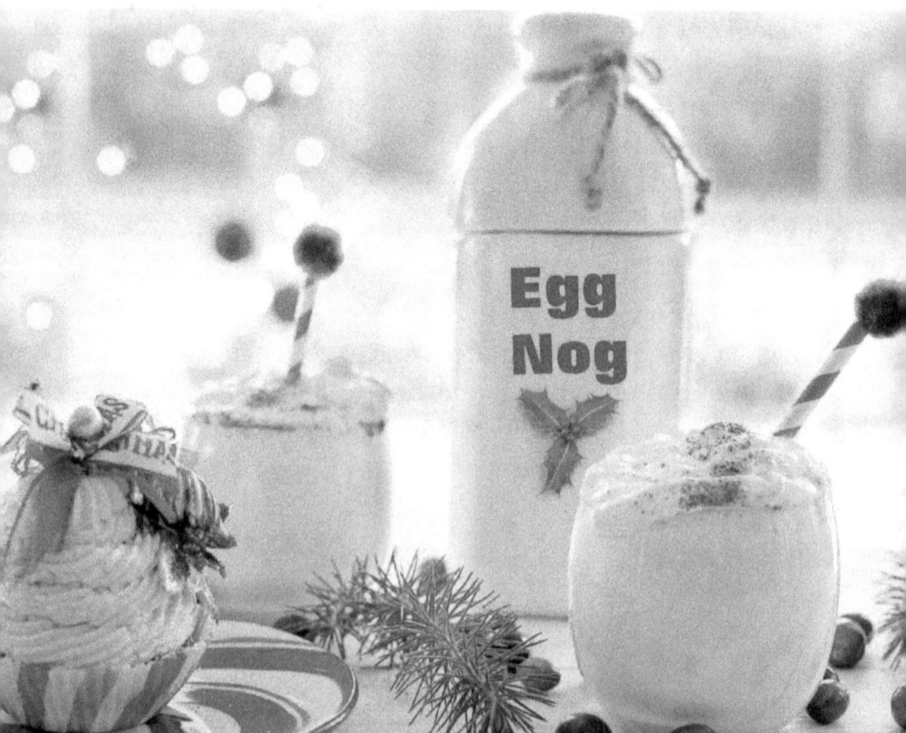

Chocolate truffles...wine...heart-shaped pizza...
conversation heart candy...there are many ways
to celebrate Valentine's Day that involve food and
drinks. But you don't have to derail your healthy
eating efforts on February 14. Here are four ways to
celebrate the holidays or a romantic occasion like
a birthday, anniversary or Valentine's Day without
busting your waistline:

1. Go for a walk or a hike. Spend some quality one-on-
one time getting some fresh air and really connecting
and talking.

2. Make a cute card for that special someone. Include
a coupon for a massage or breakfast in bed. Writing
something thoughtful is much more valuable and
precious than a box of chocolates.

3. Get a gift certificate for an experience. Whether
it's a manicure, a massage or some much-needed
babysitting time, many busy moms would appreciate
some quiet time and self-care over candy or a fancy
dinner.

Stay on Track at Parties

Whether it's a Super Bowl party, summer BBQ or other social gathering, you need to have a plan in place so you don't over eat. Always have a strategy, which includes bringing along some healthy food. Here are several ways to help you stay on track:

1. Keep your hands and mouth occupied.

It could be nursing a drink, chewing on gum, or carrying a plate and glass in your hand. Doing these types of things makes eating a little more difficult, which will help you be more conscious about what you're eating.

2. Be mindful.

Don't eat as you watch the game and don't eat as you are talking to people. When you eat, focus on eating. Whether you're munching on appetizers or sitting down to a meal, the easiest way to go crazy and lose track is to not be aware of when and what you're eating.

3. Bring a healthy option and eat before you go.

Never go to a social event starving. That is a recipe for disaster. Have a light snack to ensure you make wise choices with your head and not your stomach!

Whether you're hosting or attending a social event, bring along a healthy recipe to ensure you have options. Here are two options, one savory and one sweet. Both are easy-to-make, delicious, macro-friendly options

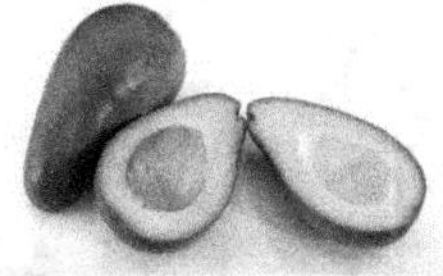

Creamy Avocado Dip

INGREDIENTS:

1/2 cup plain fat-free Greek yogurt
1 clove garlic, minced
3 tbsp. chopped fresh cilantro
1 tbsp. finely chopped seeded jalapeño pepper
2 tbsp. fresh lime juice
1/4 tsp. ground cumin
Salt and ground black pepper, to taste
Pita chips, tortilla chips, cut up veggies (for serving)

1. Place the yogurt, avocados, garlic, cilantro, jalapeño, lime juice, and cumin in a blender or food processor. Mix until smooth.
2. Season with salt and pepper, to taste.
3. Scrape dip into a serving bowl and serve with pita chips, tortilla chips, or cut up veggies.

Makes 4 servings.

Macros per serving (dip only): Calories: 133, Protein: 4.5g, Carbs: 8g, Fat: 10g

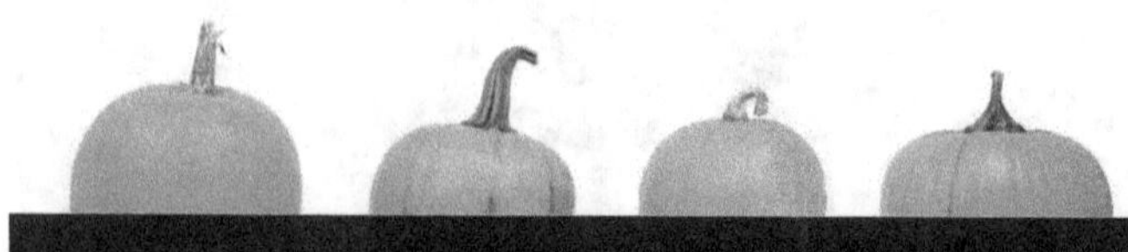

Pumpkin Cheesecake Dip

INGREDIENTS:

1 cup fat-free cottage cheese
1/2 cup pumpkin puree
1/4 cup skim or almond milk
1 tbsp. sugar-free instant butterscotch
(or vanilla) dry pudding mix
1/2 tsp. pumpkin pie spice
1/2 tsp. cinnamon
3-6 packets stevia to taste (or
sweetener of choice to taste)

Optional toppings:
- gingersnaps
- light whip cream

1. Place everything in a blender, and blend until smooth.
2. Serve immediately or cover and place in the refrigerator until chilled — at least one hour
3. Top with light whip cream and/or crushed gingersnap cookies if desired!

Makes 4 servings.

Macros per serving (dip only): Calories: 133, Protein: 4.5g, Carbs: 8g, Fat: 10g

Both of these dips taste amazing with
pretzel chips or pita chips.
Plan ahead so there are no excuses for not
sticking to your eating plan. Remember,
when you fail to plan, you plan to fail.

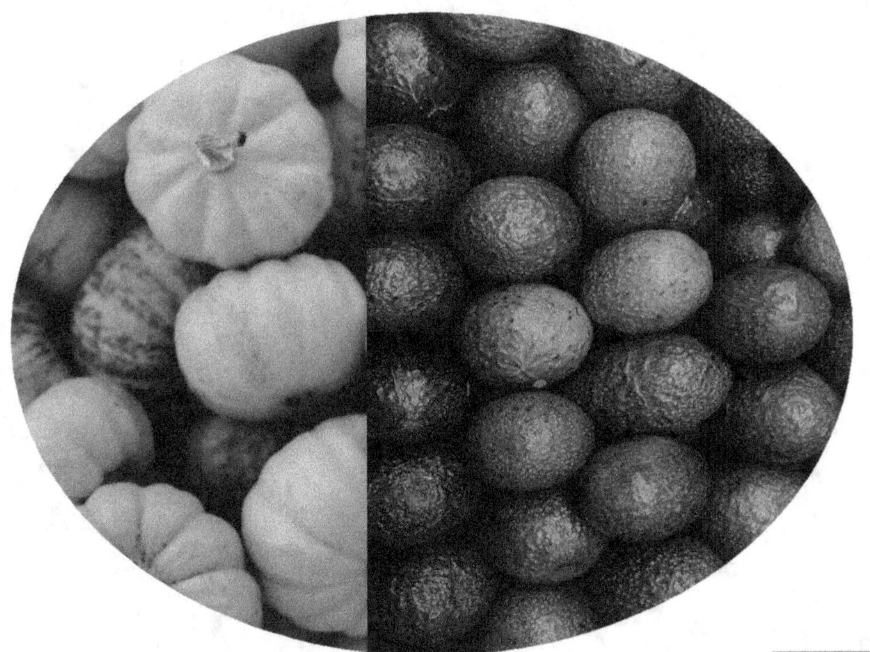

CHAPTER SEVEN

Preparing for vacation and the anticipation of going away are always so exciting! But how often do you go away, have an amazing time, but feel horrible when you return because of all of the unhealthy food you ate. Do you track how many pounds you gained or how tight your clothes feel when you come back? I know I do! But you can enjoy vacation without the guilt of gaining weight on vacation because you didn't watch your food intake. For example, I recently went to an all-inclusive in Punta Cana for five days and only gained one pound. I didn't go crazy but I did enjoy my share of beach-side drinks and decadent desserts.

Once your travel plans are booked, take a closer look at your hotel amenities. Is there a gym and/ or walking path? Are there any nearby gyms or recreational facilities? When can you get in your workouts at a time that won't disrupt planned

Staying Healthy on the Go

Whether you're traveling for vacation or if you're a corporate road warrior, planning ahead is critical to staying on track with your eating plan and workouts.

family or work activities? Then, review your food options. Is there room service or an onsite restaurant? What local restaurants are available? Are there food delivery services?

Then, you will need to pack healthy snacks and workout gear. You will want to pack snacks that are easy to get through security and will keep without a refrigerator. Having snacks on hand is great if you're flight is delayed or if you get to your hotel late at night and you're starving. Pack workout clothes and some resistance bands. If there are no gym options, you will need to work out in your room.

Being stuck at airports and hotels can mean lots of sitting and waiting. But that doesn't mean you have to sit. Take a walk around the airport, use the steps in the hotel and keep moving!

While most smart phones offer a step-tracking feature. There are a number of apps available that can help you track steps, water, food, calories and much more.

My Top Five Favorite Apps

How many times have you heard "There's an app for that?" Gotta love technology. It's simplified our lives in so many ways, including when it comes to staying in shape. With that, I'd like to share my top five favorite apps. These are the ones that I use every. Single. Day. And, they're perfect apps to help you stay on track with your fitness while you travel. Best of all, they're free, with options to pay for a premium version.

1. MyFitnessPal

As a macro-tracking ninja, this app is my go-to for logging all of my food. Plus, I'm on a 1,375-day streak that I don't want to break any time soon. The free version is perfect for most people, while I opted for the premium version at $49 per year. The paid version enables me to customize my macros, which makes my life soooo much easier. You can also customize and load your own recipes, save your favorite meals and so much more!

2. Fitbit

I'm currently on my third Fitbit device. I am seriously addicted to it. In addition to having an app on my phone, I have the Fitbit HR, which allows me to track my heart rate, see my total calories burned, steps taken and resting heart rate. Within the app you can set an alarm to have your device vibrate to wake you up, track your menstrual cycle, log your water and check your sleep cycle and time asleep. Need I say more? If you're looking for a wearable tracking device, you want to check this out.

3. Todoist

I am a to-do list junkie. If I don't have a list going, nothing is getting done. I've been using this app for nearly two years and can't imagine my life without it. It's free and allows you to keep an ongoing to-do list and assign dates, reminder and even categorize by work, personal, etc. This is so great for those on-the-go to-do's that I always seem to forget. For traveling, you can easily set reminders to pack, check in to your flight, and all of the other details you need to remember. You can also set reminders to track your food, workout, move throughout the day, and much more!

4. Strong

When I weight train in the gym, I typically use a good old pen and paper. That was until I discovered this free app. You can add weight training workouts and it includes a timer for rest periods in between sets. The best part is when it displays your personal best or personal record (PR) for exercises. Plus, it tracks how long your workout is and what you lifted during your last workout. I love being able to push and challenge myself—always shooting for those PRs! Plus, when you're on the road, you can easily create an on-the-spot workout based on the equipment you have at the hotel or resort. Just add the machines or exercises as you go. Now there's no reason not to get a good weight training workout when you travel.

5. Insight Timer

Over the past year I've incorporated meditation into my daily routine and it's been nothing short of a game-changer for me. From being able to cope with stress better to having a clearer head, meditation is where it's at. (And, we all know how stressful traveling can be.) The best part is you only need 5-10 minutes each day. This app provides a variety of options for guided meditation, or you can use their timer to do your own thing. From gratitude to stress relief, there are hundreds of meditation themes and you can bookmark them to create your own library.

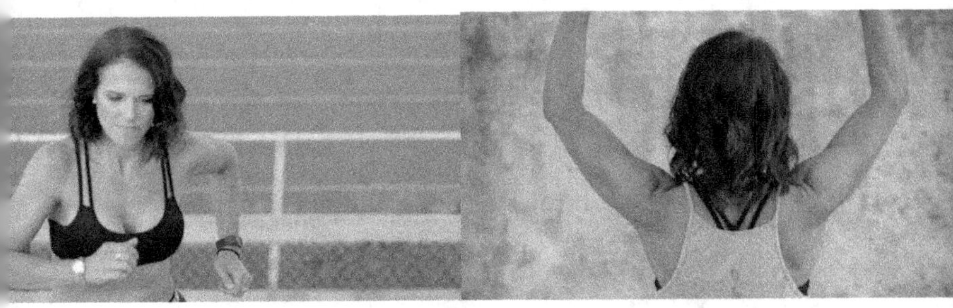

Is it consistency, motivation or something else? There are so many resources and apps available to provide support no matter what is tripping you up. From habit-tracking apps to motivational videos on YouTube, there is no shortage of information to help you. That said, it's important to have enough self-awareness to know what will help you reach your goals Is it a coach, community support or something else? Having this information will help you identify where you need help. In Chapter 10 we discuss mindset and willpower, which are critical components of any successful fitness program.

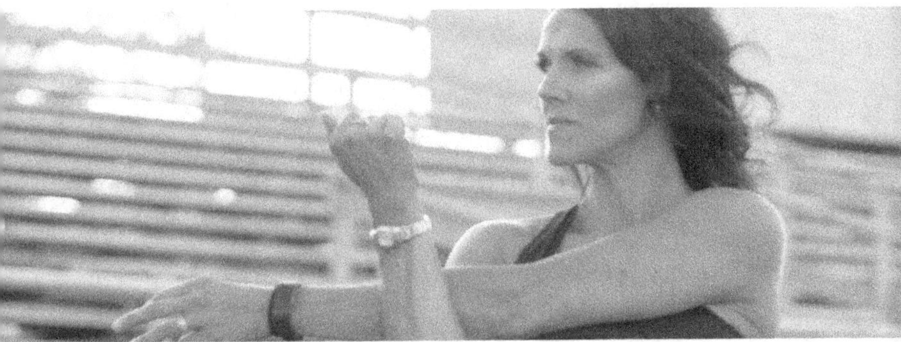

But knowing how busy most moms are with running a household and taking care of kids, our next chapter outlines ways to save time and other productivity tips when it comes to tracking macros.

CHAPTER EIGHT

Time Savers & Macro Hacks

If you're a mom, there's no question that you are busy. Whether you're a stay-at-home mom or working outside of the home, time is a commodity when you're raising children and trying to take care of yourself. I get it. I'm all about efficiency and productivity when it comes eating and exercise. Here are some helpful tips and tricks to save you time and, ultimately, your sanity:

❂ Use the barcode feature on MyFitnessPal to easily add foods to your log.

❂ Try to eat the same foods each day, then copy and paste meals and snacks.

❂ Meal prep for the week on Sundays—package all of your lunches for the week, prep all of your dinners and keep a running list on the fridge so family members can pitch in to get meals started.

❂ Always keep snacks in your purse, car and office. Never be without a healthy food option...this is what leads to diet derailments and unhealthy eating.

❂ Cook in huge batches and freeze in appropriate portions. This is a great option for soups, casseroles and vegetables.

❂ Hungry? Drink tea or coffee to subdue hunger and get you to your next meal.

❂ Veggies are so filling. If you like to eat until you are really full, make your lunches and dinners 3-4 oz lean protein and 16 oz of a green vegetable like green beans, broccoli or zucchini.

◉ Measure out and label all of your food for the week. It makes logging so much easier when you can quickly enter the weight vs. having to break out the scale each time.

◉ Add your favorite recipes to MyFitnessPal to get an accurate per-serving breakdown.

Meal Prep Time Savers

◉ Determine your menu of meals for the week, including breakfast, lunch and dinner. If you don't mind the monotony of eating the same meal for one week, I highly recommend doing that. It makes meal prep much easier.

◉ If you like to eat something different every day, you could potentially meal prep for two weeks. It will take you more time upfront, but you'll be set for two weeks and you will only need to meal prep twice a month.

◉ Do all of your food shopping on Saturday or Sunday.

◉ Spend 2-3 hours meal prepping for the entire week. This can be actually cooking everything or chopping and assembly. Do what works best for you and your family.

◉ What takes the most time? Weighing and measuring? Cutting and packaging? Set up an assembly line and do it all in one shot. You will set yourself up for a week of success.

Top Five Best Snacks for Back-to-Back Meetings

Are you often stuck in back-to-back meetings from morning until evening? Wondering when you'll get a chance to eat or even take a bathroom break? I've been there and I feel your pain! Be prepared for those crazy marathon meeting days and pack your snacks ahead of time. Here are my top five best snacks to keep on hand, whether it's in your car, your purse or your desk!

1. Hacked Snacks Protein Bites
2. Power Crunch Bar
3. Almonds + Apple
4. Quest Tortilla Chips.
5. Turkey Lettuce Wrap

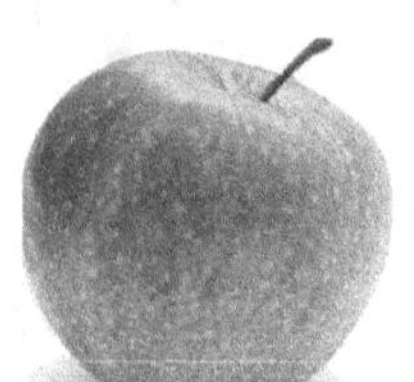

You'll notice that these snacks are low in fat and high in protein. They will help keep you full and are only around 200-250 calories. For #1, 2 and 4, there are a variety of flavors and options.

Keep these snacks on hand whether you're stuck in the car driving or waiting for a delayed flight. When you don't have options and you're ravenous, that's when bad food decisions happen!

These tips will come in handy when you're off schedule, traveling or other common monkey wrenches that are throw into the best laid plans. Being prepared and planning ahead is one of the keys to success with any program, but this one in particular. When you have your calorie and macro goals, there is not excuse to not have food handy. Today's convenience stores, restaurants and airports offer many healthy options. In addition, having food on hand in your purse, car, office and in the diaper bag will ensure you always have options.

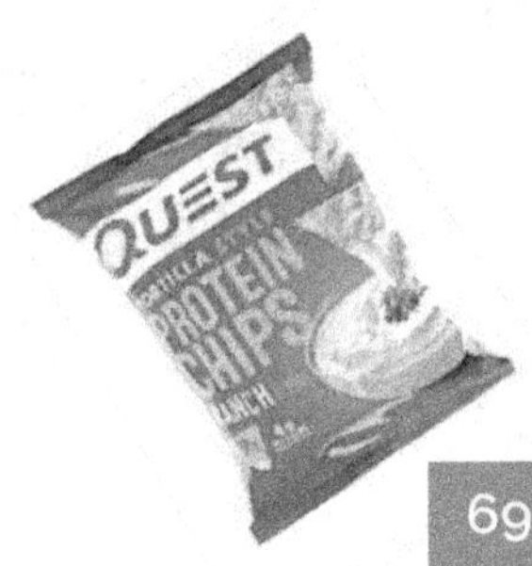

We all know that having children means schedules and priorities can change on a dime. But it's also important to enlist your kids on your healthy-eating journey and workout regime. Helping them to understand why eating right and getting enough exercise are important to leading a healthy life. The next chapter outlines how you can be a role model, and get them involved in this important journey.

Macro Kids

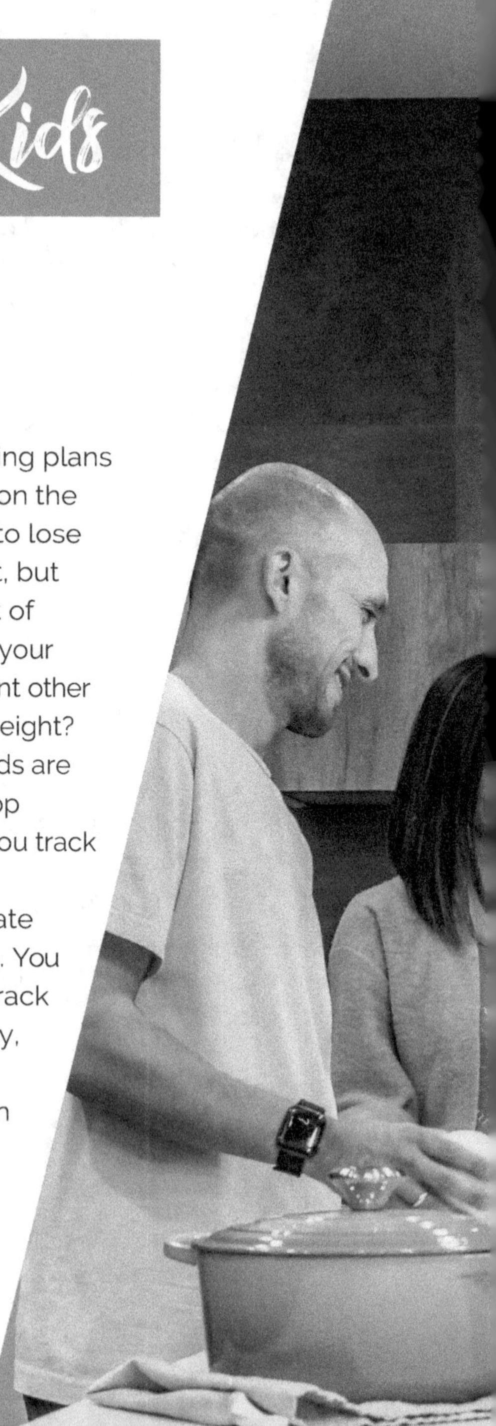

Many diets and eating plans are solely focused on the person who wants to lose weight. That's great, but what about the rest of your family? Maybe your husband or significant other wants to also lose weight? But ensuring your kids are eating healthy is a top priority, too. When you track macros there's no eat to create separate meals for everyone. You can easily stay on track and feed your family, too. This chapter outlines the solution for you.

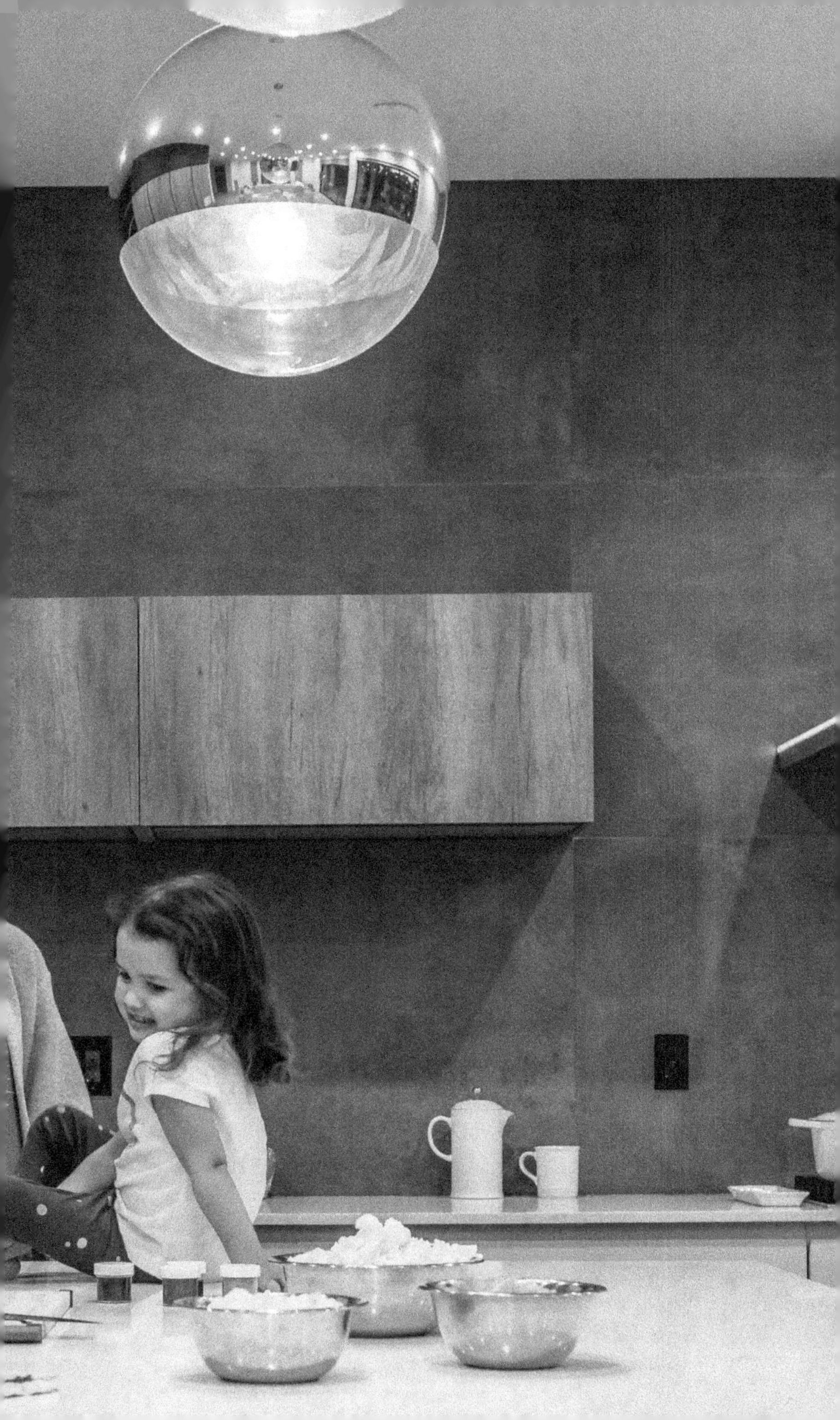

YOUR SUPPORT SYSTEM

Getting the Family on Board

As a figure competitor, my diet gets super strict as I get closer to my shows. I find that I'm normally making separate meals for my family and myself because I can't eat what they're eating.

When it comes to tracking macros and flexible dieting, you don't need to do this. Your family should be eating the same foods that you do, especially if you want them to get healthy and eat a balanced diet

Teach About Macros

So how do you get your family on board? Show them how you track, what different foods are made of (i.e., protein, carbs, fat) and help them to understand how to eat a healthy, balanced diet. One of the best ways to do this is by using MyFitnessPal, especially if you have teenagers. Have them download the app to their smartphone and track their own food. My two kids did this and were pretty shocked by the amount of carbohydrates they eat and how fattening snacks like Doritos can be versus something like yogurt.

For children 10 years old and younger, it can be helpful to explain what certain foods do and how they contribute to a healthy body. For example, how yogurt has calcium and protein to build strong bones. Or, how eating carrots can help get vitamin A (from beta- carotene) and antioxidants, which help things like heart disease.

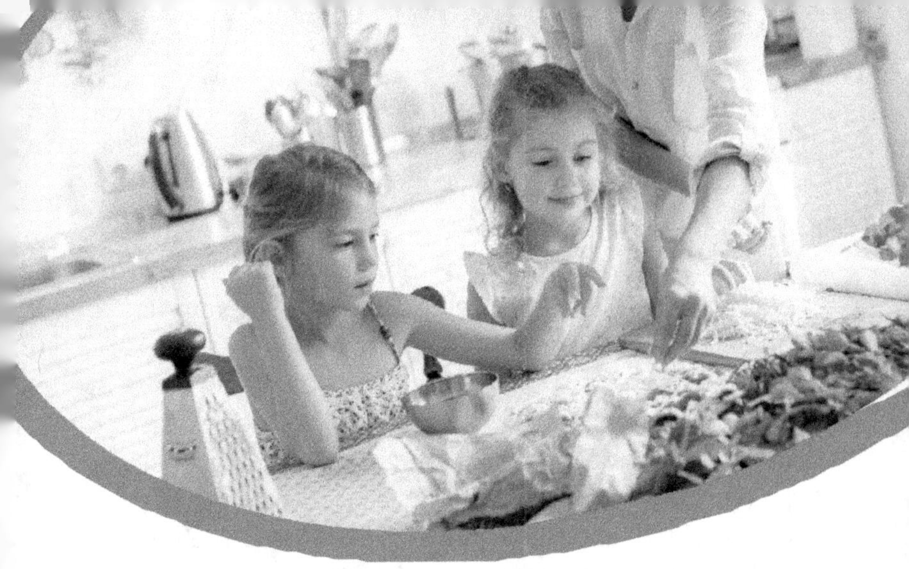

Another way to involve the kids is to explain why you prepare certain meals. For example, chicken, broccoli and rice is a healthy meal with servings of lean protein, healthy carbohydrates and the combo is low in fat. Not only that, there are a number of other nutrients and vitamins. Broccoli is a good source of fiber and protein, and contains iron, potassium, calcium, selenium and magnesium as well as the vitamins A, C, E, K and a good array of B vitamins, including folic acid. Chicken is a great source of quality protein and also a good source of thiamin, zinc, copper and manganese. Rice is a whole grain and high-quality carbohydrate that is a good source of magnesium, phosphorus, manganese, selenium, iron, folic acid, thiamine and niacin.

Helping the kids to understand the essential vitamins and minerals in healthy foods will help them to quickly begin to get on board, and in turn help you make better choices.

For example, my kids love Cheez-Its and Goldfish. These aren't horrible snacks, but they are high in carbohydrates. I try to get the whole grain version and show my kids how to add peanut butter to their snack to get some added healthy fat and protein.

Meal Prep

Kids can also help with meal prep. Instead of rushing to pack lunches during your morning routine, have them meal prep their lunch as you do yours. For example, as I prepare my lunch the night before, I ask my 12-year-old daughter to prepare her lunch, too. We talk about what healthy options are and what the different between protein, carbohydrates and fats are, as well as ensuring the lunch she packs is filling. This is also a great way to sneak in some quality time with your kids, which can be hard as they reach the pre- teen and teen years. Younger children are eager to help and will love helping mom pack her lunch.

They can also help create the weekly dinner menu. I find that when you get your children (and spouses) involved, they will begin to have a vested interest in nutrition. They'll want to understand how their favorite meals fit into the equation. For example, chicken fajitas (recipe in Chapter 4) is one of my family's favorite meals. It's a great combination of protein (chicken), carbs (tortilla + peppers and onions), and healthy fat if you add some guacamole. And, many times, you can create a healthier version of your family favorites. For example, if hamburger night is popular, use extra lean ground beef and throw in some finely chopped mushrooms, onions or other vegetables into the meat mix. Use low-carb or whole-grain rolls and low- sugar ketchup. Eating healthy doesn't have to be hard, costly or tasteless!

Many kids may balk at helping out – I encounter this scenario more often than not. It can help to turn meal prep into a game or look for ways to get them engaged. Depending upon their age, having them search for recipes on their phone or tablet can keep things interesting. You could also have them Google various foods to see what kinds of vitamins and minerals are in each one and how they benefit their body. Little will they know that they're getting a nutritional education while they're helping you!

Be Adventurous

Jump on Pinterest for a new healthy recipe or break out your cookbooks. Get your kids to pick out a new recipe to try, or find one using Google. Grab some ingredients that you have on hand and do a Google search. For example, if you have chicken breast, onions, mushrooms and tomato sauce, enter that list, add on the word "recipe" to the end and see what comes up.

With a little ingenuity, you can turn any recipe into a healthy one. Here are some additional alternatives:

- Use low-fat or non-fat cheese.
- Instead of full-fat sour cream, use non-fat Greek yogurt.
- Choose 95% lean ground beef versus 80%.
- Try riced cauliflower instead of white rice.
- Instead of pulled pork, tried pulled chicken.
- Use low-sugar or low-fat options for your favorite dressings, condiments and sauces.

One of the things I love most about tracking macros is that it's family friendly. Many fad diets like Keto and Paleo are not eating methods you would encourage your kids to do. You are a role model for your family. They are taking their eating cues from you. If you're eating vegetables, your family will follow suit. Granted this varies by age (I have teenagers that hate tomatoes while I love them).

Most importantly, depending on your kids' ages, you can begin to teach them what macronutrients are and which foods contain which macros. For example, my 12-year-old daughter and year-old son were really curious about MyFitnessPal and tracking. So, I set them up and showed them how to track and how to figure out which foods were primarily protein, carbs or fat. It was eye-opening for them to see what's in Doritos versus broccoli. That's not to say they're picking broccoli over Doritos – these are your typical teenagers! But understanding the amount of carbs in snacks compared to vegetables was a teaching moment.

Use this experience to teach your kids. Some will be interested and some will not be, but again, you are the role model.

CHAPTER TEN

Mindset is an area that is not frequently discussed when it comes to diet and exercise. But mindset is such a critically important component of your success! You will benefit from having the right mindset because it will help you when you're faced with making a decision to eat right or not eat right. It's also beneficial in understanding when you're full or if you're bored or thirsty. When you have the right mindset, you will be laser-focused on your goals and there won't be much that will deter you in reaching them. You've heard of the phrase "mind over matter." Your thoughts determine your actions. This is true whether your goals is to lose weight, start a business, run a marathon, or climb Mount Everest.

I never realized the importance of mindset until I started competing. I needed to be mentally prepared to dedicate time and effort to tracking what I ate. This is a different kind of rigor than working out because it's mental and it's a 24-hour commitment. Everything I put in my mouth had to be logged, because nearly everything contains calories.

For example, I chew a lot of sugar-free gum, at least 4-5 pieces per day. Each piece of gum has 2 grams of carbs, so chewing 5 pieces of gum meant I was consuming 10 grams of carbs. I could've had a small rice cake!

Mindset also plays a role in self-sabotage, which is a real thing. I know because I do it to myself all the time. When I get ready for a competition and start making serious progress, I suddenly start eating outside of my prep. I know it's wrong and I know the scale will reflect it, but for some reason I don't care. I think it has to do with self-worth. Am I worthy of success? Am I worthy of coming in first place? How silly does that even sound? Of course, I am! Then why would I deliberately do things to sabotage myself? Sometimes I think we are all afraid of what will happen if we are successful, especially when it comes to losing weight. What will my friends and family think? Will people look at me differently?

The most important person you need to think about is yourself. It sounds selfish, but you have your own reasons for eating right and working out. It could be for health reasons, aesthetics, to compete, or something else altogether. Regardless, that's your motivation and that's what you need to stay focused on.

How To Improve Your Mindset

There are a number of ways. Read about it, understand it, learn how to improve, or even hire a coach. Some of my favorite mindset books include: *You are a Bad Ass* by Jen Sincero, *Mindset: The New Psychology of Success* by Carolyn Dweck, and (an oldie, but a goodie) *Awaken the Giant Within* by Tony Robbins. Mindset coaches are all over social media. But be sure to do your homework and understand the coach's background, methodology and outcomes.

Talk to others who have successfully hired mindset coaches to guide them.

Mindset is tied closely to goals and motivation. The right frame of mind, having the confidence to achieve your goals and not letting stress or unplanned events will help keep you on track. How do you get into and remain in the right mindset? There are a few ways, and it will vary by person. Here's the down and dirty game plan I use to work on my mindset:

SMART GOALS

When you create goals, make sure they're **SMART**, which means **S**pecific, **M**easurable, **A**ttainable, **R**ealistic and **T**imely. SMART goals are important because it makes them very precise. You will know exactly whether or not you've attained your goal. For example, if your goal is to lose weight, you would make it **SMART** by stating it as, "I will lose 20 pounds by May 5" or, "I will work out for 30 minutes per day, three times per week."

AFFIRMATIONS

Affirmations can help you stay on track because they are a positive reminder of where your mind needs to be. No negative self-talk here. Come up with a few affirmations to help keep you on track. I have daily reminders on an app in my phone that include several affirmations:

- "My desire is stronger than my doubt."
- "Everything comes to me easily and effortlessly."
- "I deserve all of the happiness and success that I desire."

VISUALIZATION

Close your eyes and envision exactly how you want to look and feel. Picture yourself doing activities with ease, wearing clothes you've dreamed about, and feel confident and attractive.

This type of exercise is commonly used by professional athletes. Numerous studies have shown that the mental practice of focused visualization can be as effective in improving skills as real practice. Interestingly enough, when we visualize an action - whether it's working out, sticking to our diet, getting a promoted at work – the same regions of the brain are stimulated as when we perform the action and the same neural networks are created. Essentially, your brain thinks you've already completed the task at hand!

For me, I visualize winning my figure competitions. I think about how it feels to win that trophy, what it looks like from the stage, and how elated I am.

It may sound silly, but give it a try. It's as easy as daydreaming about winning the lottery – another popular form of visualization!

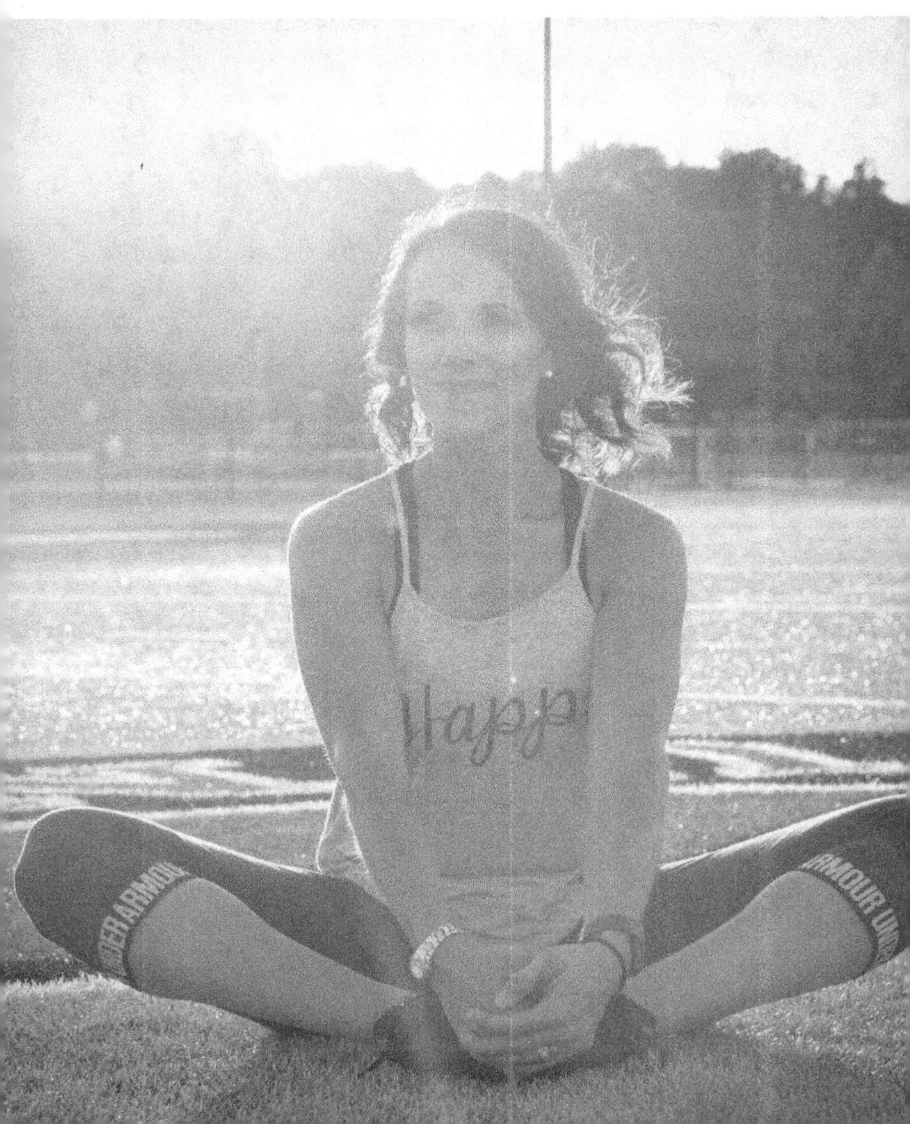

MEDITATION

Meditation was a game-changer for me. It helps clear my mind, which in turn helps me deal with stress much more effectively. It can be hard to get started and I know many people feel like they're not doing it right. I felt the same way. Meditate for 3-5 minutes each day and keep adding. I'm now at 11-15 min and I want more!! I look forward to meditation as much as I look forward to my physical workouts. Strong mind, strong body. Several apps can help you get started, including Insight Timer (what I currently use), Head Space (what I used to use), and Calm. Many people claim that meditation doesn't work for them. They can't do it; they don't know how or they can't find the time. I was the same way. Here are some tips on how you can get started and incorporate a daily meditation practice into your life.

1. Start small with 1-3 minutes of meditation.

2. Use an app and select a short, guided meditation.

3. If you prefer meditating without an app, set a timer for 1-3 minutes and sit in silence and focus on your breathing. Breathe in for a count of 4, hold for 4 counts and breathe out for 4. Repeat this process 10 times

4. Don't overthink the process. It literally means to think about nothing and clear your mind. When you do have thoughts, just realize it and let it go

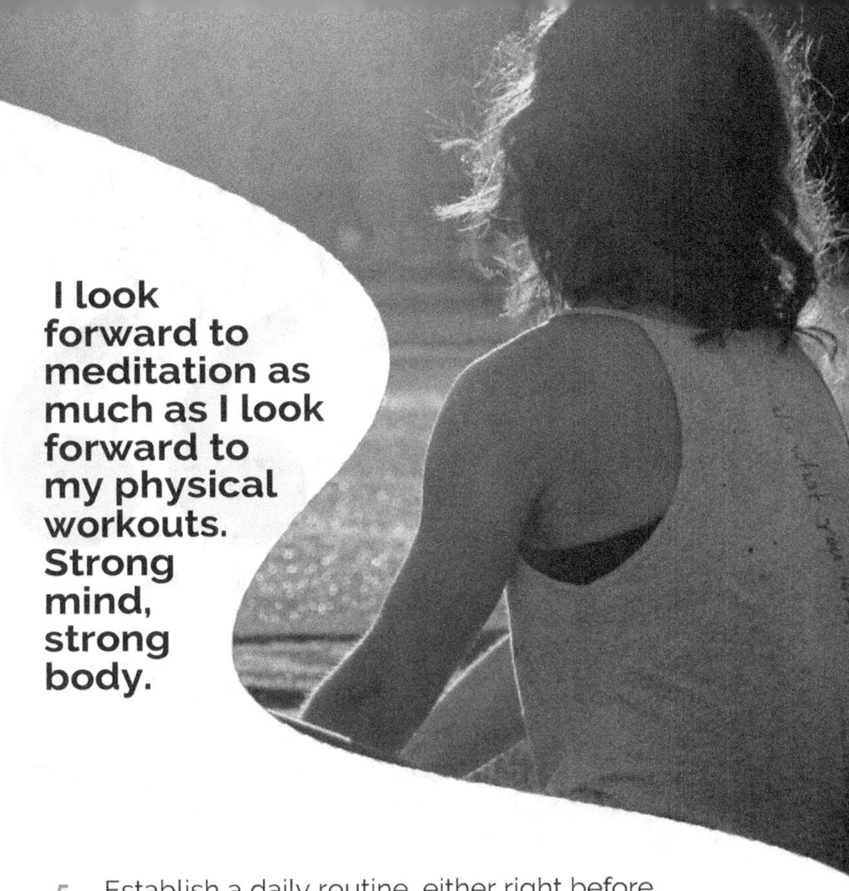

5. Establish a daily routine, either right before bed or right after your workout. Select a time that you know you can stick to and try to do it for 3-5 days in a row to get started.

6. Once you establish the habit, notice how you deal with stress and how you react to certain events.

7. For me, meditation has completely changed the way I react to stressful events. I find that I am much more grounded and even-keeled.

GRATITUDE

Cultivate a gratitude practice. I have found that having a daily practice of identifying those areas of your life where you are truly grateful can have a profound effect on your attitude and mindset. From your home and family to something as simple as a beautiful flower you saw on a walk can be part of your gratitude list. This type of practice can also help you to be more mindful and present. You will look for things to appreciate and express gratitude for, such as someone who held the door open for you or finding a heart-shaped stone.

My own gratitude practice involves journaling for two minutes each day. Here's what it includes:

- Three things I'm grateful for

- Three things that went well yesterday

- Three things I could improve

- Three top goals for the day

Why these areas? It has helped me to celebrate my successes but also note where I can improve and do better. For example, sometimes I am overly anxious or in a rush for no reason. Self-awareness and personal development are critical components of mindset as well.

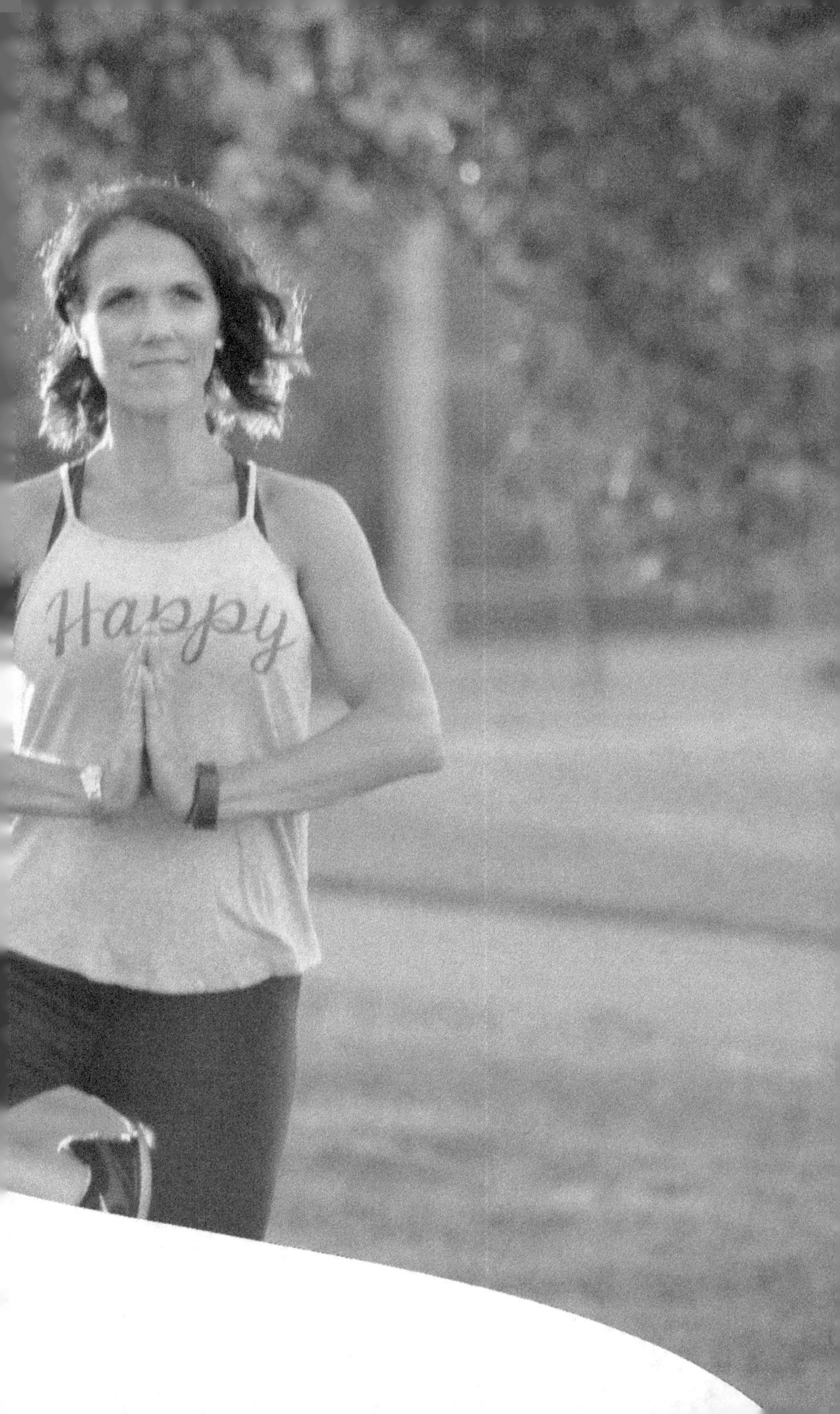
Happy

UNDERSTAND
Your Why

When it comes to self-care and losing weight, your overall goals need to go beyond aesthetics. It's not enough to fit into your favorite jeans or look good for a class reunion or wedding. Looking great in a bikini is wonderful, but dig deeper. Why do you want to lose weight?

If you're a career-driven professional, you can't rise to the top of your profession and also serve your family well without taking care of yourself. Beyond your dream body, think about your health, your energy level and your ability to take care of yourself and others.

If you're drinking five cups of coffee a day, hitting the vending machine for your meals and drinking your calories at happy hour, that is not a sustainable, healthy lifestyle. Those habits will not allow you to be your best or to function at your best. You deserve only the best, and when you begin to honor yourself and treat your body with respect, everyone around you will follow suit.

When you think about your diet and eating habits, think about fueling your body with only the best. If you had an expensive Maserati or Lamborghini, you would fuel it with premium gasoline. Well, your body is no different. It deserves only the best so it can perform at its best.

Motivation & Goals

Everyone has different goals. It could be to lose weight, to run a 5k, to exercise without back pain or to have the energy to play with your kids or your grandkids. Figuring out your "why" is critical when it comes to motivation and achieving your goals. For every goal you choose for yourself, ask "why" until you get to the true root of your goal's purpose. This will help you stay motivated and focused. Here are some examples to help you:

Goal	Why
I want to lose weight.	It will help me feel better in clothes, have more energy, increase my confidence, and reduce my cholesterol and blood pressure. I want to be healthier as I get older so I can keep up with my kids and to be a good role model.
I want to run a 5k.	I've never run more than a block and I want to see if mentally/physically, I can achieve this goal. It will help me stick with my workout plan. My spouse is a runner and it could help us become closer.

Aesthetics are nice and are an added bonus as you strive to get healthier, but they cannot dictate your goals. In addition, a number on the scale—while a great measurement and progress tool—is also not a great motivator. Instead, think ask yourself: what will losing 20 or 50 pounds do for you? I would imagine you would have more confidence. You would feel good about your body and you look in clothes. You would have more energy. From a health perspective, maybe your blood pressure goes down and your cholesterol numbers are reduced.

For many people, health and how you feel should top your list. You need to make yourself a priority. This is not an act of selfishness; this is an act of survival. It's no different than the emergency procedure on an airplane. Give yourself oxygen first and then administer it to others. The same holds true for your health. How will you be able to support and give to your family and loved ones if you are not operating at your best?

For me, competing in figure competitions keeps me accountable to my daily weight training and diet routine. It takes years to add muscle and continue to progress. I like this type of long game. Your health is a marathon, not a sprint. Finding a sustainable and flexible way to eat and exercise is critical. You won't stick to a fad diet that eliminates entire food groups, or workouts that torture you for 45+ minutes.

And, it's important to remember that everyone is different. Your goals are different and how your body operates is different. This is especially true as we age. What you could once do at 20 years old is radically different from what you can do at 45 years old. It's a battle against time. You need to keep your body operating as efficiently and effectively as possible.

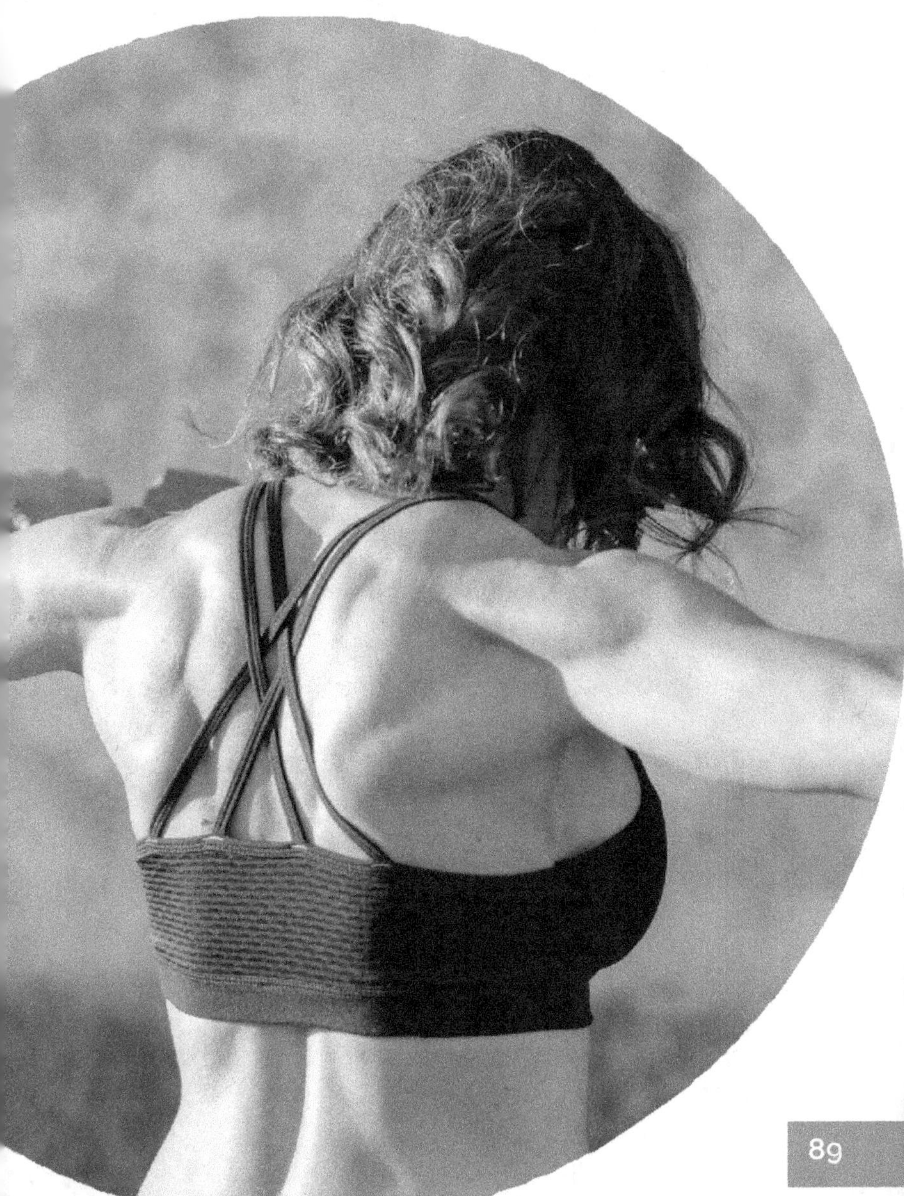

89

DOMINATE

Your Goals

There's no better time than right now to plot out your goals. When you have a clear plan of attack, it makes reaching your target that much easier.

Here are some easy-to-implement tips to help you dominate even your toughest goals:

Break Your Goal Down into Bite-Sized Segments

When you have an enormous goal like saving for a down payment on a house, running a marathon or losing 50 pounds, it's helpful to narrow down the goal to smaller steps. Look at the calendar, pick a realistic deadline and then work backwards.

Let's use losing 50 pounds as an example. A healthy rate of weight loss is 1-2 pounds per week. So, you would give yourself 30 weeks, or a little over 6 months, to lose this amount of weight. When you break a huge goal down into bite-sized segments, it becomes less scary and more attainable. Now you can break this down into 90-day, 60-day and 30-day goals. From there, you can give yourself weekly goals. Week #1 may be figuring out what diet and exercise program you will do.

Week #2 may be tracking your food and establishing an exercise routine, and so on.

Write It Down

In a September 2016 article in the Huffington Post, Dr. Gail Matthews, a psychology professor at the Dominican University in California, recently studied the art and science of goal setting. She gathered 267 men and women from all over the world, and from all walks of life, including entrepreneurs, educators, healthcare professionals, artists, lawyers and bankers. Then, she divided the participants into groups, according to who wrote down their goals and dreams, and who didn't. She discovered that those who wrote down their goals and dreams on a regular basis achieved those desires at a significantly higher level than those who did not. In fact, she found that **you become 42% more likely to achieve your goals and dreams by simply writing them down on a regular basis.**

Whether you create a list of New Year's resolutions or have just one major goal to achieve, write it down in a journal, on a Post-It that you can see every day, or hang it on your refrigerator. Take it a step further and create a vision board with images of what achieving your goal will look like.

Get an Accountability Partner

Having to answer to someone can definitely put your motivation into overdrive. Do you really want to share that you haven't made any progress towards your goal? Whether you enlist a coach or a friend, you will often go above and beyond what you set out to do to prevent having to share any kind of failure or slip-ups.

HOW TO BE

Consistent

Now that you have your goals and ways to stay on track, consistency will be key to reaching them. After countless figure competitions, I know better than most people how hard it can be to stay consistent! But consistency is the key to meeting your goals. As a working mom with a side hustle, kids, a house to take care of, and a husband, life often gets in the way. It is super easy to just sit on the couch after a long day or get an extra hour and a half of sleep in the morning instead of going to the gym. Many women often tell me that they struggle with being consistent on both fronts—diet AND exercise!

Here are a few ways to help you to be more consistent:

Make It Part of Your Routine

The easiest way to remain consistent is to make fitness part of your routine, just like brushing your teeth! You don't forget to brush your teeth, right? Well, working out and eating healthy should be as much a part of your day as brushing your teeth or your hair, or taking a shower. You don't need to be at the gym for a lengthy amount of time, or spend hours of time in the kitchen creating chef-inspired healthy meals. Keep it simple and you will be more successful in your efforts!

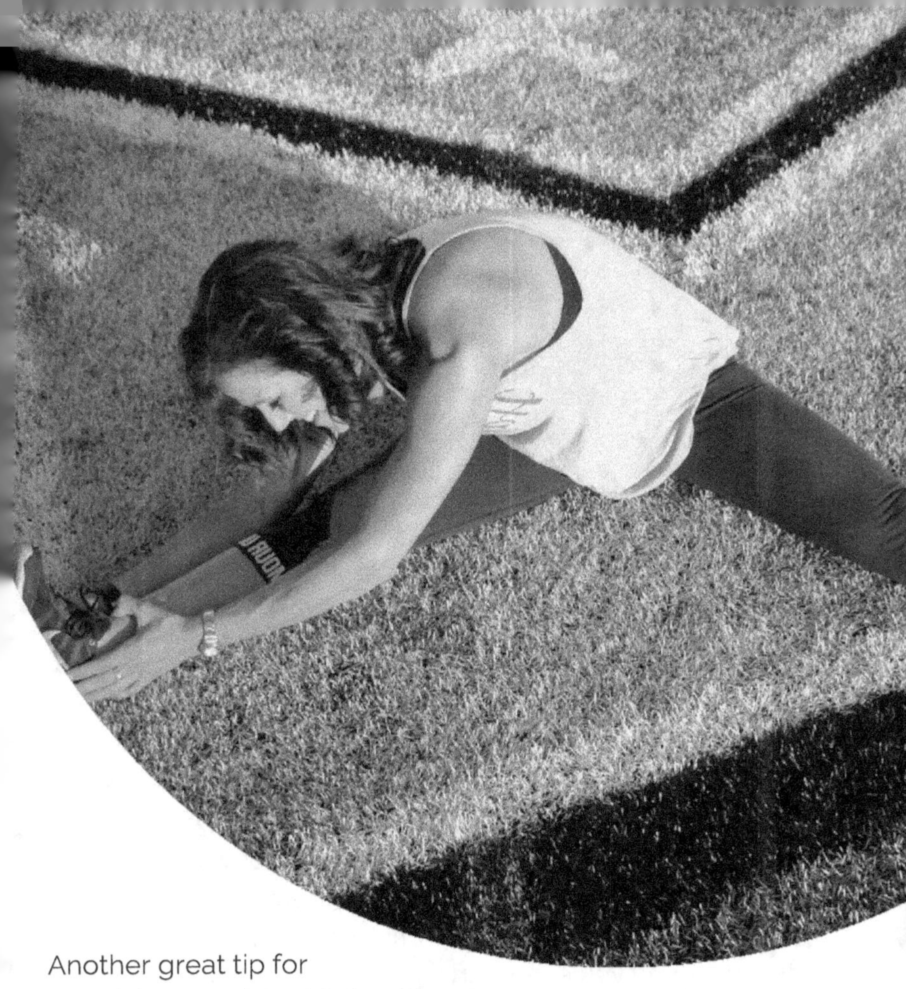

Another great tip for
remaining consistent is to either
reward or punish yourself, depending on which you prefer.
(Punish does not mean to deprive yourself of food!). A
reward can be to get a massage or a new outfit once you
reach a certain milestone. Preferably, you should stay away
from food-related rewards, since using food as a reward or
punishment can lead to incredibly dangerous habits and
disorders surrounding food relationships. A punishment
could be socking away $20-$50 dollars in savings or
skipping a nail appointment. Do whatever works for you, as
long as it is not food-related.

HOW TO BE MORE
Mindful When You're Eating

Being mindful when you eat is incredibly important. If you're not mindful, you can easily overeat, speed-eat or forget to enjoy your food. Luckily, there are different strategies you can use to ensure you are connecting with your food so you truly enjoy your meals.

Set a Timer

Don't rush through your meals. Set a timer for 15 to 20 minutes and take your time eating your meal. Chew slowly, taste your food, and enjoy what you're consuming. How many times have you eaten so fast that you barely tasted it, or finished before those around you even started? Then, you have to deal with the gastrointestinal problems that eating fast causes (e.g., gas, bloating, stomach cramps).

Limit Distractions

Turn off the TV, put your phone away and focus on your food. Look at its color, smell it, feel its texture in your mouth and use all of your senses. Make eating an experience instead of something else to check off your to-do list.

Ask Yourself: Am I Hungry?

Especially during snack time, it's important to gauge your hunger. Are you hungry, or are you thirsty or bored? Sometimes we get so caught up in "having to eat" that we don't ask ourselves, "Am I hungry," or, "Do I need to eat right now?"

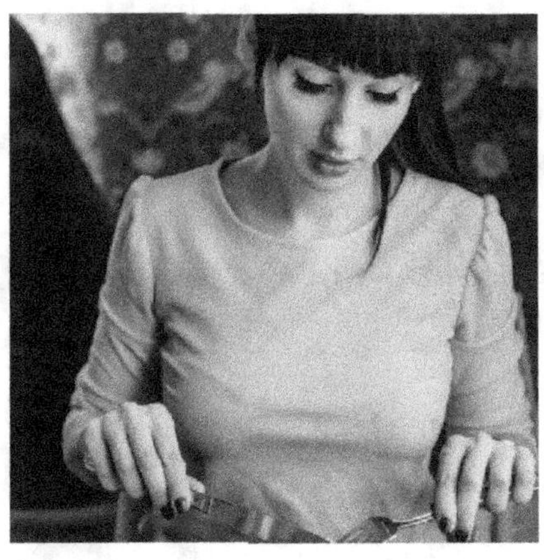

Many people use food as a crutch, so mindful eating can be helpful if you tend to binge eat, mindlessly consume food or eat to just "get it done." Enjoy your food and be sure you listen to your body.

Two occasions when mindful eating can come in handy, but can be difficult to do, is during special events, like wedding and parties, as well as when on vacation. Sometimes we can get caught up in the excitement and mindlessly eat what's in front of us. Focus on the event and the experience. When it's time to eat, focus on what you're eating. It's not easy, but it will help prevent mindless overeating, which tends to leave you with unexpected guilt and remorse. Do these sentiments sound familiar: Why did I eat all of those passed appetizers? I don't even remember what I got at the buffet. This is where mindful eating comes in. Focus on the task at hand.

HOW TO KNOW

When You're Stress Eating & What to Do About it

When it comes to losing weight, stress eating or emotional eating can quickly derail even the best laid plans.

How do you know when you're stress eating?

Typically, you stress eat when something triggers you. This could be anything from getting a rush project at work to finding out a loved one is sick. Your heart starts racing and you start searching for food. You mindlessly start putting food in your mouth without much thought to the taste or the quantity. And once you start eating, you just can't stop. We've all been there. It's not fun. But, if you plan ahead and stay aware of what you're doing, it can definitely help!

Here are a few ways to help you to be more consistent:

Distract Yourself

Creating a distraction that doesn't involve food can help ensure that you don't go off the rails on your eating plan. It can also help you destress. What does this involve? First, recognize that you're stressing out. Then, take a deep breath and think about your next course of action. Take a walk. Call a friend and spend some time catching up. Grab your workout gear and break a sweat. Pick up a book or magazine and read a few pages. Set a timer and meditate for 10 minutes. Finally, you can always pick an area of your home and start cleaning. Not only will you not be able to eat, you'll end up with a clean home!

Occupy Your Mouth

You can't eat when your mouth is occupied or minty fresh. Instead of reaching for food, reach for your toothbrush and brush your teeth. Grab a piece of sugar-free gum, candy or a low-calorie lollipop. Fill up your water bottle and start chugging! All of these options will keep your mouth occupied and hopefully keep you from reaching for food when you're not truly hungry.

Take a Moment

Nowadays everyone is constantly on the go, mindlessly looking at their phones. When you get stressed, it's important to be mindful. What does that mean? Stop and take a moment to realize that you're getting ready to stress eat and ask yourself why. Take out a journal and write a few notes about how you're feeling, the time of day and what has triggered you. You may begin to notice a pattern. Go for a walk and just talk to yourself. Say out loud what's bothering you. Sometimes when you say it, you realize how meaningless or trivial the trigger is for you. Getting to the root cause can help prevent future slip-ups.

Stress eating is so common, but you can manage it with the right mindset.

Self-Care Is More Than Aesthetics

You can't rise up to the top of your professional life and serve your family well without taking care of yourself. It's not just about looking good in a bikini...it's about your ability to take care of yourself and others, your health and your energy level.

Many people feel guilty for taking time for themselves. But if you're familiar with Stephen Covey (the author of *7 Habits of Highly Successful People)* you know he is adamant about taking time to "sharpen the saw." What does that mean? You are the saw. If you aren't taking time to recharge and invest in yourself so you can be at your best, everything else suffers. This includes your work, your business, your family, your health and more.

Are you drinking five cups of coffee a day, hitting the vending machine for your meals and drinking your calories at happy hour? Is that allowing you to be at your best? That is not okay, it's not sustainable and it's not going to allow you to rise to the next level at home or at work.

Whether your goal is to drink more water, stop smoking, eat better, get more exercise, spend more time with family, start a business or go back to school and get your degree— whatever your goal may be, taking time for yourself is key.

You deserve better...and when you begin to honor yourself and treat your body with respect, everyone around you will follow suit.

What's on deck in the coming year? Is this the year that you will make your health a priority? What will it take to get you where you need to go? Start thinking about it now, not January 1. Then put a plan into place and take action. Refer back to the goals section earlier in this chapter for tips on putting a realistic plan into place.

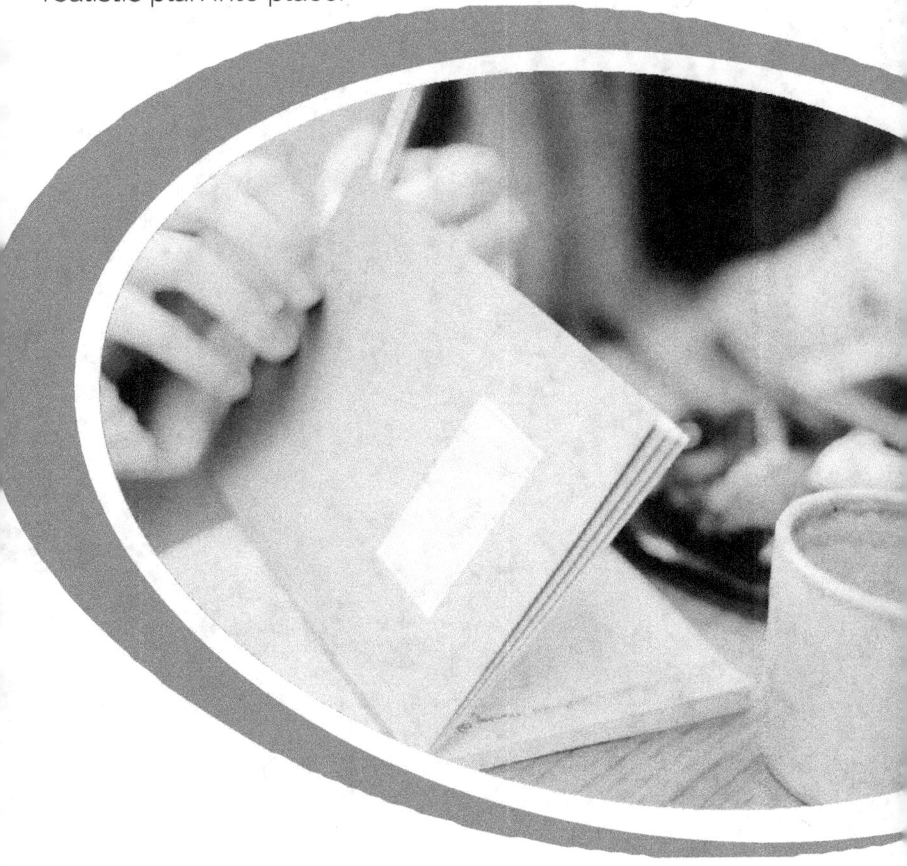

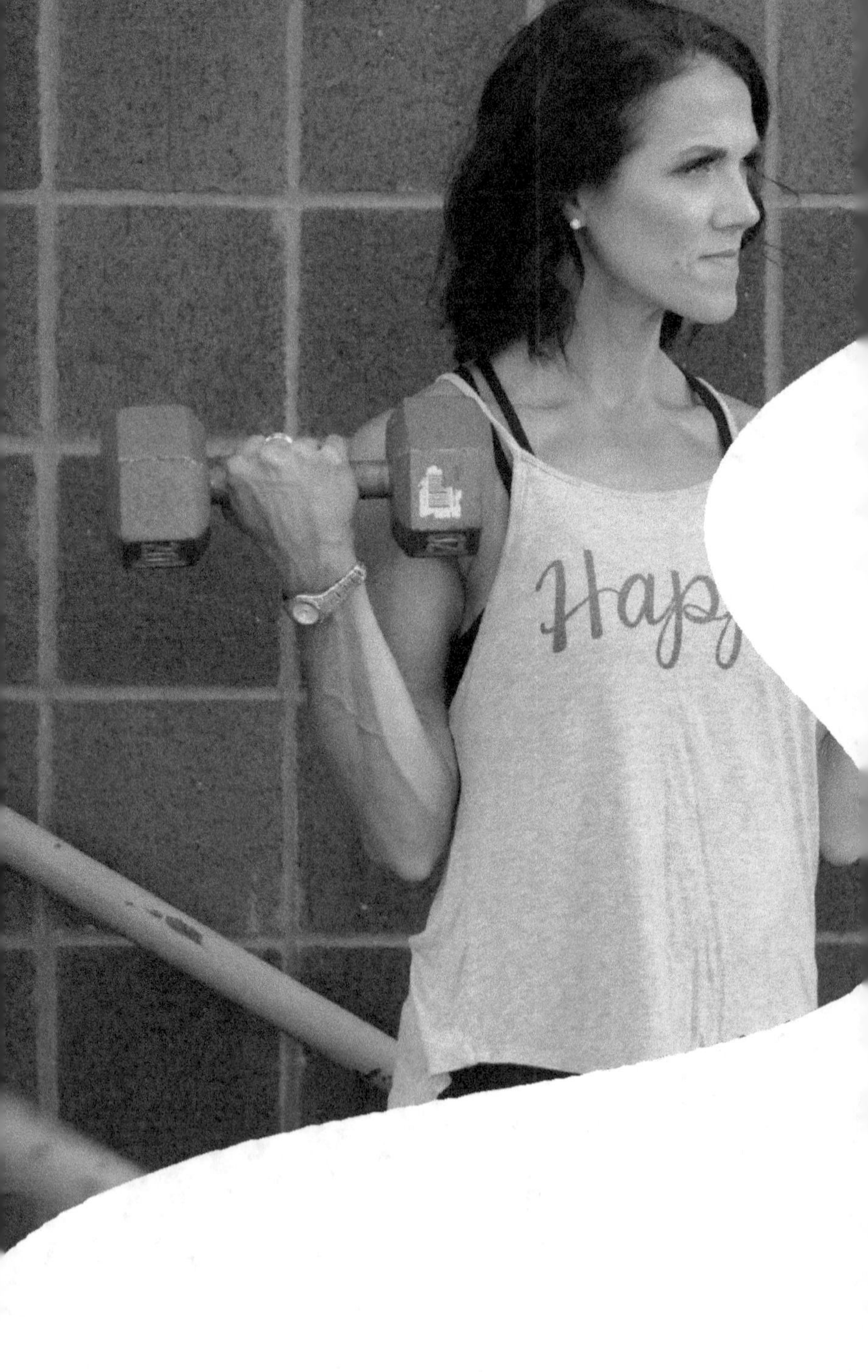
Hap

Now What?

While I hope you enjoyed this book, I truly hope you take action and implement many – if not all – of the tips and suggestions you read. Results come from inspired action. You have the tools to make changes to your body, but only you can take the first step.

I'm here for you and also have a dedicated community of women who are all working towards similar goals to yours. Come join us on Facebook or LinkedIn at Corporate Women Getting Fit. Just search for this group and join so we can help cheer you on.

We covered a lot of information so it's important to not get overwhelmed. To help you keep things simple and sustainable, make small changes each week. Here is a guide for how to use the next eight weeks to reach your goals:

Week 1 – Macros 101
- Get an understanding of macros (protein, carbs and fats) by reading Chapter 1
- Begin to read labels
- Download MyFitnessPal to your phone and start to play around with it

Week 2 – Determining Your Macro and Calorie Goals
- Review chapter 2
- Calculate your Basal Metabolic Rate (BMR)
- Calculate your Total Daily Energy Expenditure (TDEE) calories.
- Calculate your macros
- Begin casually tracking your food with MyFitnessPal

Week 3 – Start to Track Your Macros
- Review chapter 3
- Enter your goal macros in MyFitnessPal
- Begin tracking your calories and macros (everything that goes in your mouth gets tracked)
- Read labels to understand what macros are in your foods

Week 4 – Plan Ahead to Hit Your Macros
- Review chapter 4 for meal-planning and prepping tips
- Plan your dinners for the week
- Plan your breakfasts, lunches and snacks
- Create a grocery shopping list
- Shop and set aside time to meal prep

Week 5 – Outline Your Workout Plan
- Review chapter 5 for tips on creating a workout
- Determine what days and times during the week you will workout
- Write out your workout for the week (similar to how you meal prep, you want to workout prep)

Week 6 – Stay hydrated & Plan for Special Occasions
- Review chapter 6 for tips on eating out, holidays and special occasions
- Plan ahead to ensure you stay on track
- Start tracking your water and fiber

Week 7 – Keep Prepping and Tracking
- Review chapter 7 for eating on the go tips
- Continue to meal prep and track your foods
- Schedule your workouts and get them in

Week 8 – Stay on Track
- Review chapter 10 for tips on motivation and mindset
- Enlist the family's help with finding healthy recipes
- Keep tracking
- If you've lost weight, go back to chapter 2 and determine if you need to adjust your macros

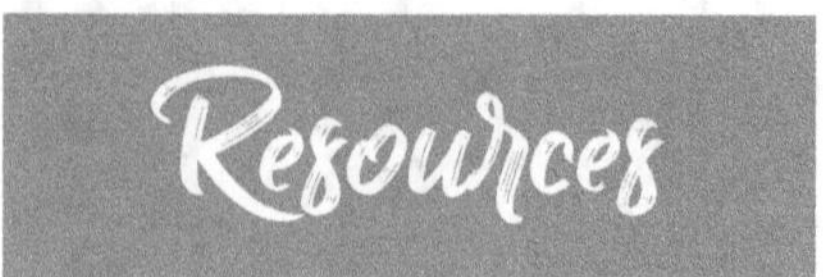

Free Bonus

Be sure to visit
www.allisonjacksonfitness.com/resources

  5-day get-lean meal plan
Beginners weight training workout
Healthy on-the-go food options
5-day meal prep healthy crockpot recipes

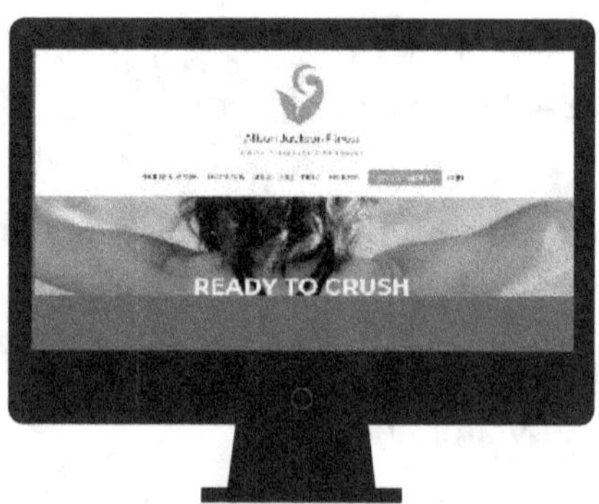

My Favorite Fitness Products...

◉ Hacked Snacks (great on-the-go protein snacks that are good for the whole family)

◉ Beverly International (my favorite brand of protein powder and supplements)

◉ DPS Nutrition (best prices for supplements)

◉ Quest (great protein bars, protein powder, protein chips)

◉ Fitbit Charge HR (I use mine to monitor my workouts, water, sleep, heart rate, menstrual cycle...I would be lost without this on my wrist each day.)

How To Measure Food Using Your Hands

YOUR HAND IS ALL YOU NEED

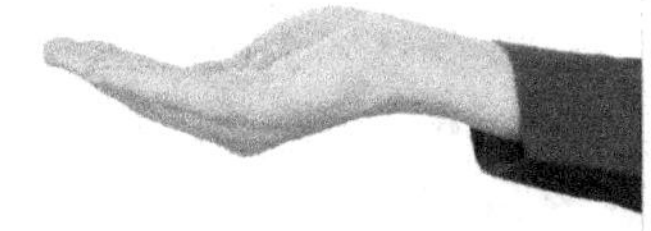

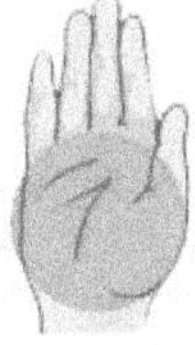

A Serving of Protein = 1 Palm

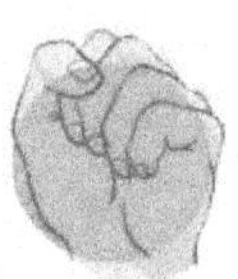

A Serving of Vegetable = 1 Fist

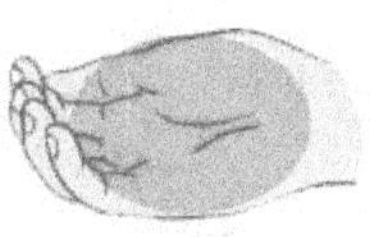

A Serving of Carbs = 1 Cupped Hand

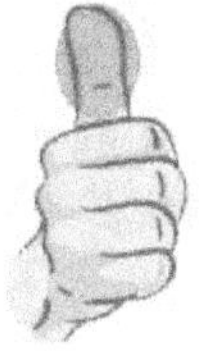

A Serving of Fats = 1 Thumb

Source:

https://www.precisionnutrition.com/calorie-control-guide-infographic

FAQ

How do I get more protein if I'm vegetarian or vegan?

There are many options to get protein if you can't eat meat. For example, seitan, tofu and many vegetables and beans have high quantities of protein, relatively speaking. Plant-based protein powders are also an option to increase your protein intake.

When should I change my macros?

As you hit plateaus and stop losing weight, you'll want to go back and reassess your macros using the calculations in chapter one. Frequently, you may need to tweak your macros slightly and/or slightly reduce your calories. However, also be sure that you're being honest with yourself. Are you tracking accurately? Those little tastes and bites here and there add up. They can also stall your weight loss. Before you make changes, take an honest assessment of your efforts.

How do I know how much cardio to do?

For general heart health, you should include at least two cardio sessions per week that can be either steady state or high intensity interval training (HIIT). For fat loss, start with three sessions and evaluate your progress each week. Before adding cardio, ensure you are truly hitting your macros and try to incorporate weight training into your exercise routine.

What is the best cardio?

The best cardio is the cardio you enjoy doing. The type of cardio does not matter; the quality of your workout is what matters. Choose whichever machine or activity that works best for you. From walking to the elliptical to spin classes, incorporate whichever cardio you enjoy most.

I love bread. What are my best options?

Carbs are not the enemy, including bread. If you're watching your carbs, choose low-carb options. Ezekiel bread is very good and there are many light varieties.

I hate protein powder. Do I have to use it?

No, there is no rule saying you must use protein powder. It can be difficult to get enough protein in your diet and protein powder can help. However, whole foods work just fine, too. Do what's best for you.

Can I eat fruit?

Yes! The reason tracking macros is called "flexible dieting" or "If It Fits Your Macros" is because you can have anything, including fruit! That said, you may be watching your carb intake. If that's the case, here is a list of carb-friendly fruits:

- ✔ blueberries
- ✔ raspberries
- ✔ strawberries
- ✔ blackberries
- ✔ kiwi

- ✔ honeydew
- ✔ plums
- ✔ nectarines
- ✔ apples
- ✔ pears

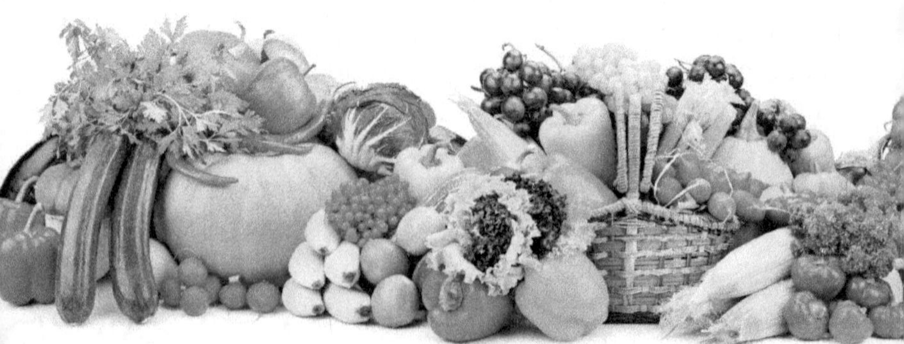

Nothing is off limits

You just need to be cognizant of your portions.

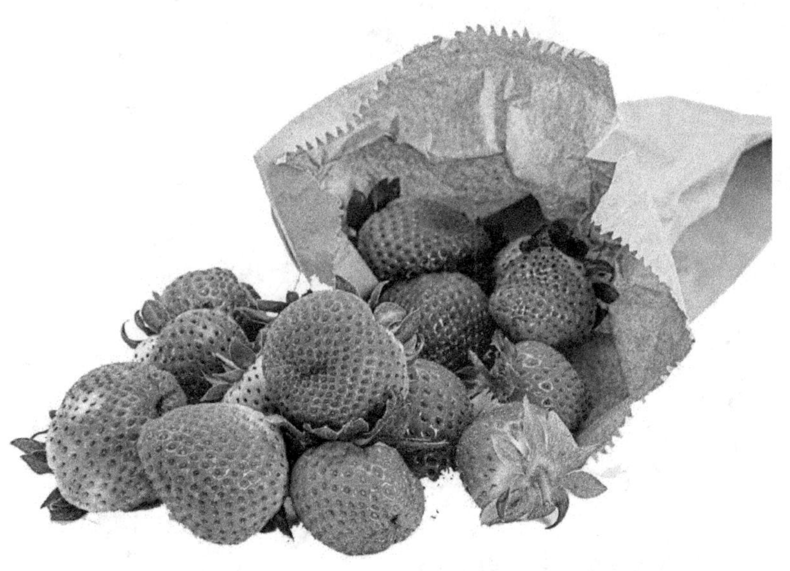

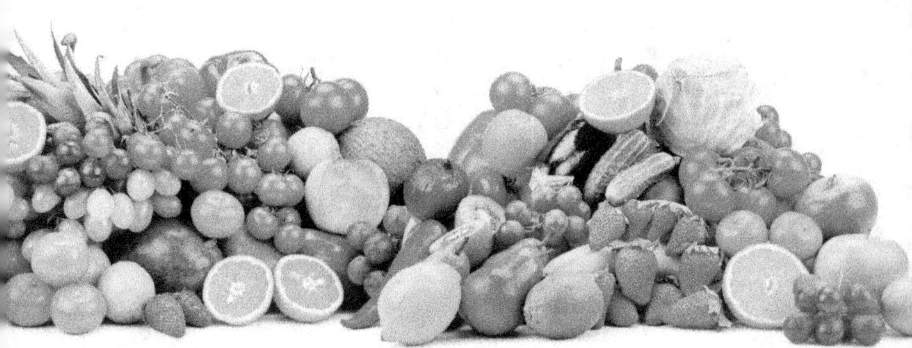

Breakfast

DAY	PROTEIN (GRAMS)
SUNDAY	
MONDAY	
TUESDAY	
WEDNESDAY	
THURSDAY	
FRIDAY	
SATURDAY	

CARB (GRAMS)	FAT (GRAMS)

Lunch

DAY	PROTEIN (GRAMS)
SUNDAY	
MONDAY	
TUESDAY	
WEDNESDAY	
THURSDAY	
FRIDAY	
SATURDAY	

CARB (GRAMS)	FAT (GRAMS)

DAY	PROTEIN (GRAMS)
SUNDAY	
MONDAY	
TUESDAY	
WEDNESDAY	
THURSDAY	
FRIDAY	
SATURDAY	

CARB (GRAMS)	FAT (GRAMS)

APPENDIX A

10 Excuse Busters

If you have excuses, I have solutions! As a coach, I see so many common excuses for not being able to eat right or workout. So, I've compiled the top 10 excuses I see with an action plan to overcome it. Use these excuse busters and you will be well on your way to a fitter, healthier self as you kick those excuses to the curb!

Excuse 1: I have no time.

Everyone gets the same 24 hours in a day. What you do with those hours is entirely up to you. If being healthy and in shape is a priority, you will find the time. Make appointments with yourself just as you would a meeting or doctor appointment. Most importantly—show up!!! Be accountable to yourself. No one is going to do it for you.

Action

Go to your calendar (online or paper) right now and schedule 20 minutes to work out on Monday, Wednesday and Friday. Select the time that works best for your schedule, whether it's first thing in the morning, during your lunch hour or after dinner. Make it simple: walk. Nowhere to walk? Here is a simple workout plan you can do anywhere:

DO 10 repetitions of each exercise these, before moving on to the next one. Repeat until you hit 20 minutes.

1. Jumping jacks
2. Squats
3. Push ups
4. Crunch
5. Lunge
6. Jumping jacks
7. Plie squat
8. Crunch
9. Push up

Take a water break and repeat.

Excuse 2: I have no money

Determine what workout works best for your budget. It could be as simple as investing in good sneakers for walking or running.

Action

Go to your calendar (online or paper) right now and schedule 20 minutes to work out on Monday, Wednesday and Friday. Select the time that works best for your schedule, whether it's first thing in the morning, during your lunch hour or after dinner. Make it simple: walk. Nowhere to walk? Here is a simple workout plan you can do anywhere:

Excuse 3: I have no motivation.

Having a bad day? Lose your exercise mojo? Just not feeling it? When it comes to motivation, you need to dig deep and ask yourself why you want to work out and eat right. It may be to feel good, prepare for an upcoming special event or because you need a change. No matter what your reasoning, you need to have a burning desire that will keep you focused and moving forward. Take some time to think long and hard about why your health is important to you. Is it about being about able to keep up with your kids? Do you want to try competing in a 5k or triathlon? Or, do you just want to feel good about yourself?

Action

Put pen to paper and list your top three reasons for wanting to eat right and exercise. Take this list and post it where you will see it each and every day, whether it's on your bathroom mirror or on your fridge.

Excuse 4: I don't know what diet/workout to follow.

There are so many diets and exercise programs available, it can be hard to know where to start. The best plan of attack is to take baby steps, plan ahead and try to be consistent. For starters, eliminate as much processed food and sugar as you can. Don't drink your calories.

Action

Most importantly, eat healthy food that you enjoy and follow an exercise program that is fun.

Being healthy shouldn't be tortuous.

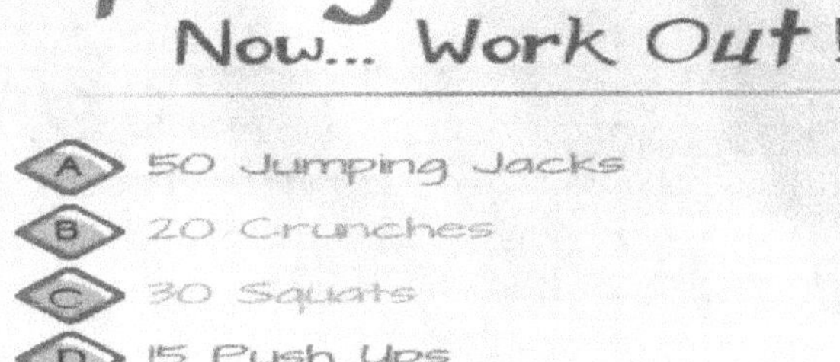

Spell *your* Name
Now... Work Out !

- **A** — 50 Jumping Jacks
- **B** — 20 Crunches
- **C** — 30 Squats
- **D** — 15 Push Ups
- **E** — 1 Minute Wallsit
- **F** — 10 Burpees
- **G** — 20 Sec. Arm Circles
- **H** — 20 Squats
- **I** — 30 Jumping Jacks
- **J** — 15 Crunches
- **K** — 10 Push Ups
- **L** — 2 Minute Wallsit
- **M** — 20 Burpees
- **N** — 40 Jumping Jacks
- **O** — 25 Burpees
- **P** — 15 Sec. Arm Circles
- **Q** — 30 Crunches
- **R** — 15 Push Ups
- **S** — 30 Burpees
- **T** — 15 Squats
- **U** — 30 Sec. Arm Circles
- **V** — 3 Minute Wallsit
- **W** — 20 Burpees
- **X** — 60 Jumping Jacks
- **Y** — 10 Crunches
- **Z** — 20 Push Ups

REPEAT 2X

Excuse 5: I don't have the space/equipment needed to workout.

You don't need fancy equipment or a gym membership. If you have your body weight, you have enough to get a solid workout. On page 119 is an easy, quick workout that you can do anywhere -- in a hotel room, in your living room, etc. You'll also find a great at-home workout in Chapter 5.

Action

Try the spell-your-name workout or walk for 15 minutes each day, gradually increasing to 30 minutes each day. It doesn't have to be 30 consecutive minutes, either. You can do 10 minutes in the morning, 10 at lunch and 10 after dinner. Spreading it out will also stoke your metabolism!

Excuse 6: I hate exercise.

What do you hate about exercise? Is it the sweating? Do you feel uncoordinated? Figure out why you have a negative association with exercise, then figure out a work-around.

Hate to sweat? Walk at a brisk pace so you're winded but not sweating. If you feel uncoordinated, don't take that Zumba class or try climbing onto the elliptical. Go for a walk, march in place or grab a bike.

Action

Find an activity that you enjoy and find fun. Jump rope, boot camp, inline skating, mountain biking...do that for   10 minutes each day, gradually increasing the time to 30 minutes. Before long, you'll wish you could workout longer!

Excuse 7: I hate vegetables and healthy food.

With so many recipe options available, it's easy to find ways to make vegetables and other healthy foods taste amazing. Don't force yourself to eat plain broccoli or bland chicken breast. From crockpots to stir-fry meals, there are countless ways to create delicious, healthy meals.

Action

Pick two of your favorite recipes and find ways to make them healthy using the tips you learned earlier in this book. For example, can you bake it instead of frying?

Excuse 8: I have an injury.

Depending upon what your specific injury is, there are ways to cautiously work around it. For example, if you hurt your ankle and it's difficult to walk, swimming or the stationary bike may be good alternatives. If walking or running is completely out of the picture, using weights for your upper body or floor exercises like Pilates or yoga may work for you. Most importantly, consult with your doctor and take it easy. Working out with an injury is a good way to hurt yourself.

Action

Consult with your doctor and follow his or her instructions. Don't ignore pain or discomfort.

Excuse 9: I have no support from family or friends.

No one can be responsible for your success but you. While it would be nice to have your own cheering section, that's not always the case. That said, you can enlist some outside support if needed.

Action

Find an accountability partner. A great way to do this is to join a Facebook group that focuses on getting into shape. There are hundreds out there. Or if you belong to a gym, see if you can find a like-minded partner with whom you can periodically check-in.

Excuse 10: I'm too old, too fat, too thin, to short, too tall, too rich, too poor.

There are a million excuses to not do something. But remember, everyone has the same 24 hours each day. It's what you prioritize as important that gets the most attention. Eliminate your excuses before they can interfere. Take control today!

Action

List every excuse you can think of and put an excuse buster next to it. Plot out how you will incorporate exercise into each day. Start small and build slowly. Consistency and sustainability are your keys to success. You got this!

Notes

Afterword

As with many people, one of my lifelong dreams has been to write a book. Never in my wildest dreams did I imagine that I would write a book on health and fitness. It's like a dream come true.

What I shared in this book is much of what I've learned over a lifetime of dieting, working out and helping others. I wanted to provide a forum for those who aren't comfortable online or who enjoy having a reference that they can hold, mark up and keep handy. There's nothing like a good old-fashioned book.

While having a book full of useful information is great, taking action is key to making changes. If you find that you're still struggling and you want and need accountability and extra support, I'm here for you. You can reach me by visiting www.allisonjacksonfitness. com. I currently offer one-on-one and group coaching—all online and virtual—so you can be located anywhere and I can still help you!

I always love hearing feedback and would love for you to send me a note on Instagram, Facebook, LinkedIn or your favorite go-to social network— @allisonjacksonfitness — especially if you've found success using the info in this book. Nothing makes me happier than helping others reach their goals.

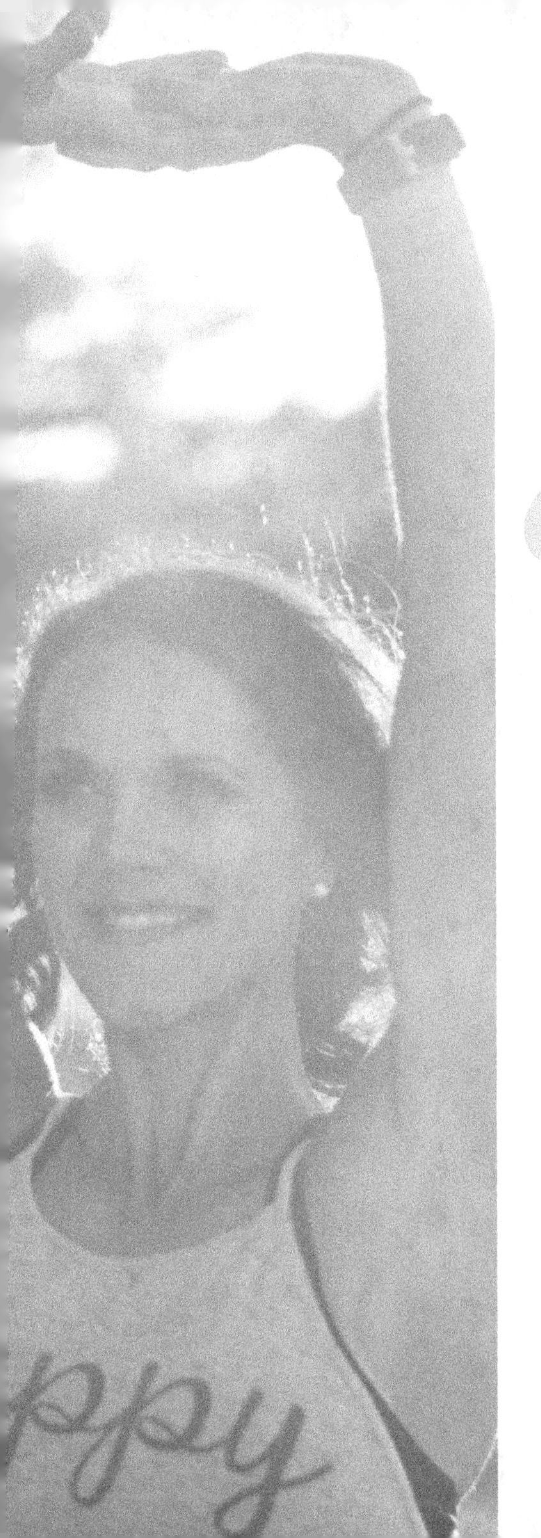

> Here's to your health, happiness and crushing your goals, no matter how big or small!

www.ingramcontent.com/pod-product-compliance
Lightning Source LLC
Chambersburg PA
CBHW070843250726

48662CB00003B/1338